TH
THAT AWAY FROM ME

Compiled by

Jackie McGregor

D1556397

'The song is ended, but as the songwriter wrote,

The melody lingers on'

Quote from 'They Can't Take That Away from Me'

by George and Ira Gershwin

Published by Accent Press Ltd – 2011

ISBN 9781907726965

Typeset and design by Jamie Russell

Printed and bound in the UK

Cover Design by Lisa Walsh

This book is dedicated to the memory of my late mother Christina McGregor and my darling father John McGregor.

ACKNOWLEDGEMENTS

Sincere thanks to the following people:

Hazel and Bob Cushion for taking this project on with such enthusiasm, also Alison Stokes and all at Accent Press.

To each one of the celebrities who have contributed. Thanks for your kindness and taking the time to help with this project. Also to all of the agents, managers and PAs who made it possible, with a special thank you to Anna Kerslake.

An enormous thank you goes to a special lady, Rhian Cowburn, without whose help this book wouldn't have contained such fabulous names. I will always be amazed by how kind you were to a stranger, Rhian, you have a huge heart (despite what the surgeon says!) and I thank you from the bottom of mine. You're a star!

To Paul Allen, Celebrity Liaison Officer for The Alzheimer's Society, who fulfilled my every request for help.

To all of the amazing Staff of Dunanney Care Home, especially Margaret Sloan, Farah Vergara, Geraldine McAuley and John Taplin for his music therapy. Thank you everyone at Dunanney for caring for dad.

To my husband Steven Guy (my rock), thank you for putting up with all my madness, you have my heart always. And to my son Ben, the most amazing and precious gift I have ever received, your love has been a healing balm to my heart.

Thanks to all of my family, especially to my brother Roy McGregor and my sister Kay Williamson, for their support and my good friend Ann McKenna.

To Sheila Leadbetter and Bruce Bovill who encouraged me through my darkest days and to Sandra Chapman for all her kindness.

To Marie Thompson who saved my sanity, God bless you Marie.

Thank you to the little band of lovely, generous-spirited, author angels for all of your advice, help and support particularly Adele Parks, Margaret James, Milly Johnson, Trisha Ashley, Belinda Jones, Sue Moorcroft, Christina Jones, Jill Mansell, RJ Ellory and Joanna Trollope.

Finally, thank you to the Almighty Invisible Hand that has guided me throughout, I commit this work to you for success.

Foreword

I have always found it easy to remember words of songs because they are put to music. I would not remember them if they weren't, as in a poem. It's something to do with the rhythm and spacing of the words in time with the music, just like children learning nursery rhymes.

Music has been a wonderful gift in my life. It is a powerful, evocative force capable of blowing the dust off our memories and taking us back to a particular place or a certain time instantly.

This book is a collection of musical memories of well-known people who have kindly donated a memory to help those with Alzheimer's disease. The editor hopes this book will raise much needed funds for The Alzheimer's Society. I hope you will enjoy reading it.

Dame Vera Lynn DBE

Messages of Support

Prince William has asked me to convey to you his heartfelt sympathy for the difficulties that you face as a full-time carer. It is truly heartening to learn that in the midst of the pain of watching your father suffer from Alzheimer's, you have determined to do all you can to raise awareness of this dreadful disease.

His Royal Highness has asked me to send his best wishes to you and your family.

From: The Office of HRH Prince William of Wales and HRH Prince Henry of Wales

His Holiness appreciates the important role music and the arts play in human society, for they provide us ways to communicate certain ideas and attitudes. When used positively, they serve as powerful opportunities to foster peace and the growth of fundamental human qualities like love, compassion and forgiveness. From that point of view your plans for the book are admirable.

His Holiness sends his prayers and wishes for the success of this project.

From: The Office of His Holiness the Dalai Lama

With our best wishes for your endeavour.

Wishing you every success with your book and with your efforts to raise money for the Alzheimer's Society.

His Royal Highness has asked me to say how very sorry he was to learn that both of your parents had been afflicted by Alzheimer's. The Prince of Wales has asked me to pass on his very best wishes.

Shakespeare said, 'If music be the food of love, play on!' and no one can argue with Shakespeare! This book is an act of love. Do read it.

From Adele Parks

Alzheimer's disease is a shameless thief of time that stole precious and irretrievable years from my mother and her family. Music was a huge part of her life before the illness took hold and it provided an invaluable bridge through the mist between us in her latter years. The music was always there for us all, an unmistakable link between reminiscence and reality. My thanks to Jackie McGregor for her wonderful work in raising awareness and funds for this dreadful disease.

From Rick Guard

Songs can be a wonderful reminder of a loved one or a special occasion so I was delighted to contribute, especially as the proceeds will be donated to Alzheimer's Society. My mum had Alzheimer's, so I know how devastating this disease and its impact can be – not only on the person who has been diagnosed but also on their family and friends. It's a cruel disease which gradually robs you of the person you know and love. The funds raised through the sales of Jacqui's book will make a difference to the lives of people with dementia and their families.

From Lynda Bellingham

Alzheimer's Disease is a cruel deterioration of a person's mental and physical health. The person afflicted gradually forgets everything they learned from childhood to adulthood including the very basic activities. It is a living hell for those with the disease and heartbreak for their loved ones. My mother had Alzheimer's disease for seven years. I watched her disappear as the woman I knew into a helpless, confused person not cognisant of her situation in the later stages. This disease is affecting more and more people, especially as the population's life span is increasing. I would like to see greater research into preventing and controlling it.

From Lynsey de Paul.

As someone who has known and helped to care for people with dementia, I'm well aware of the beneficial effects of music. Just hearing a much-loved song or tune can brighten a sufferer's day, and bring some much-needed sunshine into a clouded life. The royalties raised through the sale of this book will go towards making still-precious lives worth living.

From Margaret James

I have a number of friends whose parents have suffered from Alzheimer's so I know how devastating it has been for them to watch someone so close not be able to communicate with them. The fact they are unable to respond no matter how much love and care you give them makes it truly heartbreaking. I do hope Jackie's book will help towards one day finding a cure for this dreadful disease. I heartily endorse it.

From Denise Welch

My mother had Alzheimer's. Conversation with her had become impossible, yet on a car drive one day she sang every song word-perfect to a Frank Sinatra CD.

Music seems to have an effect on this illness.

From Sir Michael Parkinson.

My mother had Alzheimer's for so many years before being diagnosed and music certainly helped me cope with her disease.

From Britt Ekland

Introduction

My mother Christina died five years ago. She had an intense love affair with my father John for 58 years. Then a monster stole into her brain and changed her for ever. We fought it in every way we could but we lost Mum. This monster is commonly known as Alzheimer's disease. In a cruel twist of fate the disease attacked my father following my mother's death, the first thing it did was rob him of his speech, an especially brutal act of theft as my father was a such an orally competent man, described by all as charming and, above all, a gentleman. He is now confined to a silent world. I don't know what goes on behind those once beautiful, sapphire blue eyes until a chord from a song is played and he begins to weep. The song is Moonlight Serenade, which was my parents' special tune. They often talked about dancing beneath the mirror ball to this refrain in The Plaza Ballroom in Belfast, a place long gone but apparently not forgotten, even by a man with Alzheimer's, as he is magically transported back to that place of his youth, with my glamorous mother in his arms, on the strings of a melody that lingers on in his heart.

My father had been a professional musician and orchestra manager. He had his own band called the J McGregor Orchestra and they blasted out big band swing in the dance halls of Northern Ireland during the 1940s, 1950s and 1960s. His hero was Glenn Miller; dad even took to wearing spectacles with plain glass in them just to look like Miller. However, he didn't need spectacles the night he first laid eyes on my mother. It was across a crowded dance hall. Their eyes met and he knew immediately she was the one. He asked her to dance and, several hours later, he proposed. In the coming months Mum and Dad were married; she gave up the chance to go to American after winning an X-Factor style singing competition, the prize was to travel to the USA and make a record, she married Dad instead, such was her love for him. It was a union to last a lifetime for my mother and produced four children.

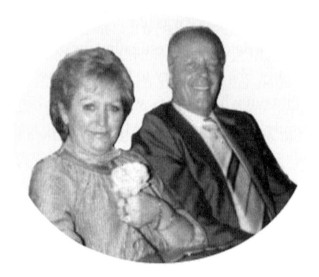

There are currently 750,000 people with dementia in the UK. The financial cost of dementia to the country is over £20 billion a year. Family carers of people with Alzheimer's save the country £6 billion a year, but the cost to their own health, both physically and mentally is beyond estimation.

My father and I looked after my mother at home. Personally, it was one of the darkest and most difficult periods of my life. There were times when I felt I was going to go insane, it was 24-hour care. We had to remove the mirrors from around our home because my mum's reflection terrified her, she no longer knew her own face. She thought she saw rats sitting on the chairs and frequently spoke in what sounded like a foreign tongue. I had to keep the doors locked and carry the keys at all times, as she would attempt to get out to 'go home' every day. My mother's existence was like a Columbo mystery, each day she became a detective investigating the disappearance of her own identity. She would try to fit together what evidence she had to find out who she was, where she lived and who on earth the family around her were. My mother no longer knew that I was her daughter or that my father was her husband and constantly waited on her long dead mother coming to collect her. 'When's my mother coming to get me?' was the refrain my father and I repeatedly listened to on a daily basis. There was no explaining to her that her mother was dead, we tried once and she screamed in grief and pain, we had to call a doctor, such was the state she was in, she forgot all about it an hour later.

The aspect I find hardest to accept with this disease is its ability to wipe out its victim's love for someone. My mother forgot that my father was the love of her life. One night she even threatened to call the police for him when he told her he was her husband, claiming he was an impostor; she had no memory of him, their marriage or their life together. It was around this time that I began to see the sparkle of my father's brilliant blue eyes begin to fade as the light of his life dimmed.

Apart from one brief time, Mum never remembered or accepted again that Dad was her husband ,which made our living routine in the house nightmarish sometimes. It was like being in a horror movie. I watched my father being with the woman he loved all day yet never being able to communicate with her or love her as his wife. I wanted my mother back so much and sometimes couldn't bear to be in the same room as my 'hologram' mother. The stress got to me and I began to have panic attacks. I became agoraphobic. Life was torturous.

Then Mum took a chest infection, one of many. She had suffered from a lung disease called bronchiectasis since I was a child. She was admitted to hospital and developed pneumonia there. We spent almost three months sitting at her bedside. One day my father walked into the ward and my mother shouted his name 'John!' it was amazing, he ran to her and held her in his arms, the relief on his face that she had come back to him almost broke my heart. He held her close, she was desperate to let him know that she knew he was there, it was as though she had been held prisoner in her body and couldn't get past the Alzheimer's monster within to be with Dad. 'I love you, I love you, I love you John,' she managed to get out. The effort took every bit of fight she had in her. I have never witnessed anything so amazingly touching and in that moment my heart filled with pride for my brave little mother for bypassing the demon for seconds and in those moments, she was steadfastly determined she was not leaving this world without telling my daddy one last time that she loved him. Just days later my mother passed away, but for my father her monumental effort to come back to him through the mists of this vile disease was everything he needed to survive.

Five months after my mother's death I married my first love, on 19 August 2005 at 3 p.m. The following year, on 19 August 2006 at 3 p.m. our son was born. My father adored him, they bonded immediately, we all lived together as a happy family for a while, but Dad wasn't himself.

My father's speech had become impaired when my mother died. After a visit to the doctor it was decided that Dad's speech problem was a grief-induced condition, he had always been in excellent health and never been to a doctor, he was now 80 years of age. Life became difficult again, getting used to being a wife and mother, keeping my writing going and dealing with an ever-increasingly reliant father. Dad had become like Mum and stuck by my side 24 hours a day. He couldn't bear to be away from me, Mum had been just the same, this proved to be very stressful.

One morning I watched him making his porridge, a daily occurrence for years, and he simply couldn't do it. He began to forget more and more how to carry out the easiest tasks. I heard alarm bells ringing in my head but ignored them.

Dad was a very healthy man. I couldn't face the thought that Alzheimer's might be a possibility, because as far as I was concerned I could tolerate anything except having to deal with this monster again. But sure enough it had come back for us. After a brain scan in 2008 just 2 days before Christmas, I was informed in a phone call that my father had 100 per cent Alzheimer's (my mother had vascular dementia mixed with Alzheimer's). I put the phone down in a daze, looked at my toddler and wondered how the hell I was going to cope. As it turned out I coped well for over a year looking after my father 24/7, seeing to his personal care and being with him at all times while tending to my child and battling my agoraphobia and panic, but it is impossible for one person to keep up this level of care. My father would wait outside my bedroom door most of the night, he slept little and just wanted to see me at all times. I dreaded having to get up to go to the loo in the night as he would think it was morning and wanted to be showered and dressed. I eventually had to get help from carers who called in during the day to help with personal care. Mentally and physically I was going downhill fast, so was Dad, he didn't even know how to turn a door knob to open the door. I was so exhausted I performed my daily tasks like a robot, I had no feelings, I couldn't afford to have them. If I thought too much I would simply go mad. I had grown to hate Alzheimer's with a vengeance, it had become my nemesis, this fight had become personal. Then my son and I both caught a nasty virus. I could barely stand. As I attempted to make lunch my knees gave way beneath me, I fell to the floor with no energy to get up.

I lay there looking at my boy and I knew this life I had been living was no longer possible. I needed a break. Fortunately I had a fantastic social worker, Marie Thompson. She had been trying to persuade me to put Dad in respite for a while but I wouldn't hear of it. I phoned her and explained the situation, she found Dad a respite place for the next day, (I owe her my sanity).

I lay awake all night crying and feeling sick, how could I let him go? I had never been without him. I packed his bag and explained that I wasn't well and he was going to have a few days in respite care, he smiled and patted me on the shoulder. I saw heartache in his blue eyes which was reflected in my own, but my father's love for me was still there and he knew I wasn't coping. I watched him get into the special taxi. Never in my life have I ever experienced such pain. My heart physically ached, I could barely breathe and I felt like I had committed a horrific crime. It was, to date, the worst day of my life, I will never forget the agony I felt.

As the days went by I got a little stronger and began to see what life was like not being a carer, which I had been to my mother most of my adult life. Dad seemed content in respite. When I phoned to see how he was, one of the nurses, Farah Vegara, asked had Dad ever played the piano? I said no, but he had been a professional musician, drums being his instrument. Farah said that John Taplin, a nurse in the home, had been carrying out music therapy with the residents and my father had mimed playing the piano and had then begun to cry when he heard Moonlight Serenade. It became clear that music was evoking memories of Mum for him. I suddenly had a vision of my mother singing in the kitchen, at the top her voice, 'They Can't Take That Away From Me', one of her favourite songs, and I thought it remarkable how there were memories of Mum that simply couldn't be taken away from Dad. Yet for her, it was memories of her mother that couldn't be erased.

I sat that night thinking about Dad and the effect the song had. I'd heard that The Alzheimer's Society had been giving music therapy to patients in Belfast with good results. According to research, listening to favourite tunes of one's past evokes vivid memories that appear to be immune to Alzheimer's. By making a soundtrack of songs that are special to a sufferer (much like the one author Adele Parks has made in this book) and then playing it back to them regularly, it could help form a resistance to this disease. Songs cause a mental movie to play in our heads and we may see quite clearly a much-loved and lost face. Sir Thomas Beecham said; 'Magical music never leaves the memory' and that appears to be true even in the case of those with Alzheimer's. Unfortunately the funding for the therapy ran out in our region. I wondered if there was anything I could to do to raise money for the Alzheimer's Society to help them carry out their important work, including funding music therapy. I felt terrible for not being able to look after my dad and needed to find a way to at least help others, this disease had left me feeling helpless in the years I had dealt with it, I needed to fight it some way. If we could help others then maybe the terrible suffering my mother had gone though and father was still going through wouldn't be entirely in vain. Then the idea came to me. I could ask celebrities what song evokes a special memory for them and put it into a book to raise money. It was a mad plan. I knew nothing about contacting celebrities nor how to get a book published, but the first publisher I contacted, Accent Press, liked the idea. I began to get replies from celebrities, Paul O'Grady and Dame Judi Dench being the first to respond. This project was going to be possible! And here it is. A book where celebrities have given a memory to help those who have lost theirs through Alzheimer's disease.

My father struggles on valiantly. I miss him so much. I miss his wonderful, entertaining, charming company and the way he could make me ache with laughter with his observations of the world. I've always been proud of my father, he's the sort of man who makes you want to stop people and shout that's my dad! No matter where I had to go or what I had to do, my father was always there supporting me. His hand was never far from mine. Whatever the future holds, I have a lifetime of love and memories that Dad and I have shared to carry in my heart, and I know that guiding hand of his will remain forever on my shoulder. I never once thought that he wouldn't be there, as naïve as that seems. You don't, you see, you never think in the midst of blissful normality that things will ever change, that this person whom you love, who has always been there, might not be any more. None of us seem to fully grasp or understand life's fragility until it's too late. And so Dad and I continue to say our long goodbye.

I wish he and my mother could be aware of this book and the kindness of strangers who have wanted to help fight this disease after hearing their story. They would be so touched. I tried to explain to Dad about the book and he looked at me with tears in his eyes. I have no way of knowing if he understood and was moved, or if the illness was simply torturing him. It's a vile disease, research and care regarding it are severely underfunded. We need to find more ways of fighting it.

I'd like to thank all of the kind-hearted people who have contributed their special memories to this book and you the reader for buying it. I hope you enjoy this musical memory tour, the royalties of which will go to help those with Alzheimer's disease.

Jackie McGregor

Professional UK lady wrestler

Danny Boy

I lost my beloved mother in June 2008. I didn't visit often because I was then and still am living in Weymouth, Dorset. Until I moved there I saw her every day maybe only for 10 minutes, sometimes for hours. We would laugh so much, she swore like a sailor and was an enormous gossip but I loved her so much. She would talk about her days in Ireland where I believe she was most happy in all her life living "in sin" with her toy boy Danny Donaghey.

She was always proud that I'd become a professional wrestler and when we were on tour in Ireland, usually with a team that consisted of 'Giant Haystacks' and lots of the old World of Sport wrestlers she would welcome all of us. All the time crowds would be gathering outside her house as Giant Haystacks caused a stir wherever he went and Mum would feed around 15 of us at a time for a wonderful meal (salmon that had been caught fresh that morning by Danny himself). Our promoter was a great man called Orig Williams who also is sadly no longer with us. He would eat his meal then insist they'd have a song and of course he'd begin to sing 'Oh Danny Boy' and he made us all sing along. It always made my mother cry. I loved those trips to Ireland. We often did shows

1

for the army out there; our British troops were constantly on alert as it was a bad time of bombings and war, not a nice place to be when things went wrong but the people I met were salt of the earth and they'd give you their last. Amazing people.

Those days long over and Mum back in our native home of Stoke on Trent, we often reminisced of those times. You could see she wished she was still there.

I lost Mum to a heart attack. I got a phone call from my son's dad who lived in America no one over here could bring themselves to tell me she'd gone. I don't think I'd ever felt such pain as I did that moment knowing she'd passed away. I raced up the motorways to get to Stoke, that 250 mile journey seemed like an eternity. Finally I saw her at the hospital, laid in the chapel of rest and I begged her to look at me and tell me she loved me but she'd gone and I'd never got to say goodbye or to tell her all the times that I'd argued with her and been mean to her, been too outspoken and disrespectful that I never meant it that I loved her with all my heart.

The day she got buried the sun shone and the church was absolutely packed which was a testimony to how well she was loved. Lots of my wrestler friends were there to support me and I'll be forever grateful for their kindness. Mum wasn't religious at all; in fact she was downright blasphemous but funny with it! I knew what I wanted to hear at my mum's funeral as did my sisters and as they carried her in Eva Cassidy sang 'Oh Danny Boy'. I thought my heart would break. I cried until I had nothing left and the rest of the service went by in a haze.

Two years have passed now and I often think of my mum and the pain is no longer sharp but the loneliness of being without her still is. Every time I hear that song I always cry wherever I am or whatever I'm doing, and that for me is my most powerful music memory.

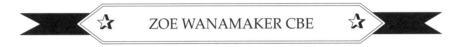

☆ ZOE WANAMAKER CBE ☆

Actress

The Overture from La Traviata

There's no particular reason except – I just start to cry as soon as I hear it.

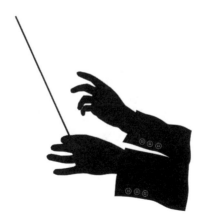

TV presenter

As Time Goes By

One of my favourite countries in the world is Portugal. We have a house in the Algarve and our summer family holidays provide us with some wonderful memories year after year, particularly because my husband Neil's birthday is in August while we are there. We always have a party and often go down to a beach restaurant beside the Atlantic later on. When we get home we put on Rod Stewart and dance on the terrace under the stars. Our favourite song is 'As Time Goes By', we play it at least once and whenever I hear it on the radio driving my car when we are back in London, I am reminded of those lovely moments in Portugal.

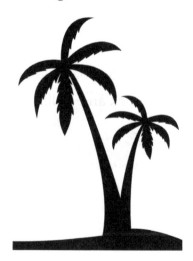

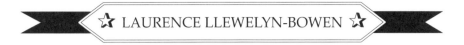

LAURENCE LLEWELYN-BOWEN

Interior designer and TV presenter

Stand and Deliver by Adam and the Ants

The song 'Stand and Deliver' by Adam and the Ants evokes memories of the hedonistic wild 80s for me, when men were men and dressed like women.

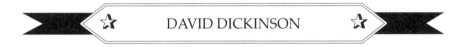

DAVID DICKINSON

TV presenter and antiques expert

Rock Around the Clock by Bill Haley and the Comets

'Rock Around the Clock' brings back youth, great times, girls, fun and of course, Rock and Roll!

Actor, theatre director and author

Caro Mio Ben by Giuseppe Giordano

Many songs have been with me all my life. One of the earliest I remember is 'Caro Mio Ben' by Giuseppe Giordano, an eighteenth century Italian composer. It's an unforgettable little love song. I was taught it by my music teacher whom I loved, Doris Bamford. I next heard it sung by Beniamino Gigli, live in concert. (It's pronounced JeelYee not Jeely) Some years later I bought an LP called 'Italian Classical Arias', sung by Gigli, and there it was again. If you're going to listen to it, that's the one to hear. It's old-fashioned singing; gorgeous and immaculate. The words are few, and simple. 'My darling love, without you, my heart aches. Believe me, I've about had it with this agony!'

I introduced my wife Kara to it and she learned to sing it, to my accompaniment. Then my daughter came along and when she was four or five, I recorded her singing it. I'm about to play that recording to my grandson, Arthur, in the hope that he'll sing it. As I write this, the birth of my second grandchild is imminent so I hope to add that voice to the collection.

Listen. You won't be disappointed.

6

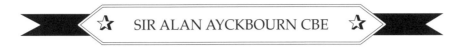

SIR ALAN AYCKBOURN CBE

Playwright and director

Lay Lady Lay by Bob Dylan

Bob Dylan's 'Lay Lady Lay' which my partner and I played incessantly – for obvious reasons. It worked. Dear Reader, I married her.

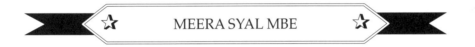

MEERA SYAL MBE

Actress, comedienne, writer

Dream a Little Dream of Me by Ella Fitzgerald and Louis Armstrong

If I had to choose one song it would be 'Dream a Little Dream of Me' sung by Ella Fitzgerald and Louis Armstrong, as it brings back memories of a wonderful trip to Australia and of falling in love while there.

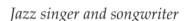

Jazz singer and songwriter

I Was Born Under a Wandering Star

Mum was a hardworking, endlessly busy housewife with four loud and demanding children to cope with. She hardly ever got time to sit down and simply enjoy time for herself, reading or listening to music. The majority of her entertainment in my early years seemed to come from Radio 4, a smorgasbord of The Archers, Desert Island Discs and of course (legendary in our household) The David Jacobs Show. She adored, what was to me, 'old time music'. I was told on a regular basis that 'this is real music' and 'they don't write them like this any more'. Now I'm in my 30s I've got to agree with her. There are countless classics that I can hear and visualise her singing along to, while seeming to simultaneously wash, iron and prepare a meal for a family of six! From 'Come Fly With Me' by Sinatra' to 'Ave Maria' (she loved anything religious). However, her crowning glory and finest comedy performance of my youth was without doubt 'I Was Born Under a Wandering Star' from the film *Paint Your Wagon*. It was a never-ending source of joy, to hear this rather 'proper' wonderful woman, with a natural soprano voice and a love of classical music, turn on the charm and perform a rip-roaring rendition of Lee Marvin's signature song in the lowest bass voice I've ever heard a female produce.

This is a delicious memory of my childhood, but what makes it so special to me is that in the last year of her life when the cruellest of diseases that is Alzheimer's had a full grip on her senses, I only had to utter a few notes of this tune and 'the lights' would momentarily switch on. She would appear transported, lifted out of the fog. She'd smile, attempt to sing along and wallow again in her silly little song. Some of those days in her last year, I'm sure she had no idea who I was, or where or who she was, but for a few moments that song would bring us back together, as we always were. The power of music! For her, and for that, I am eternally grateful.

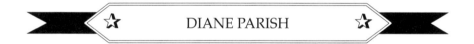

DIANE PARISH

Eastenders actress

Someday We'll All Be Free by Donny Hathaway

An evocative song for me is 'Someday We'll All Be Free' by Donny Hathaway.

Singer

Me Olvidé de Vivir

The song 'Me Olvidé de Vivir' ('I Forgot to Live') has a special significance to me. Its lyrics are about the precious moments in our lives, which we usually don't learn to cherish, until it's too late.

When I was 20, I had a car crash, which left me semi-paralyzed for a year and a half. The doctors were telling me that I would never walk again, but life was very generous and gave me a second chance. During those months, in the hospital, I understood that we should never take things for granted, we should treasure everything we have and enjoy each moment.

'After running around in life, without braking,
I forgot that life lasts one moment,
After wanting to be the first at everything,
I forgot to live the small details.

After running around to gain time from time,
Wanting to steal sleep from my nights,
After so much failure, so many attempts
For wanting to discover something new every day.

I forgot to live, I forgot to live …'

Extract of the Song: "Me Olvidé de Vivir", translated from Spanish into English.
(Authors of the song: Julio Iglesias / Manuel de la Calva / Ramón Arcusa / Jacques Revaux / Pierre Billon / M. Díaz / M. Korman / J. Flores)

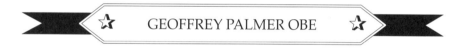
☆ GEOFFREY PALMER OBE ☆

Actor

La Vie en Rose by Edith Piaf

'La Vie en Rose' sung by Edith Piaf for me will always bring back vivid memories of the late 40s and early 50s and early holidays abroad, the distinctive smell of Gauloises, garlic and French loos. France, Italy, Spain they seemed to be playing it everywhere. A wonderful, evocative song. The man said, 'Strange how potent cheap music is', well, if this is cheap, let's not bother with the expensive stuff!

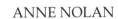

Author and singer, former member of the 'The Nolans' group

Ave Maria

Firstly I'd like to say that this book is a wonderful idea, and I am both touched and honoured to have been asked for my input.

I have chosen a piece of music which is incredibly close to my heart as it always makes me think of my mum. The song 'Ave Maria' is very special to me in lots of ways. My mum sang it at my wedding, and at my brothers' and sisters' weddings. She taught me to sing it, and then like her I sang it at many weddings, and also at my uncle's funeral. But what makes this whole experience even more poignant for me is that I then went on to sing it at my mum's funeral when she died from the affects of Alzheimer's in 2007. Ave Maria will always remind me of Mum.

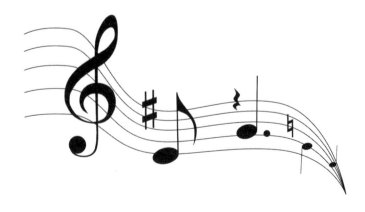

TV presenter, journalist and author

American Pie by Don McLean

My song is 'American Pie' by Don McLean, which was a global hit in 1971. It evokes strong memories of my 15-year-old self. I had learned to play acoustic guitar and my friend Paul Dedman, also an aspiring guitarist, and I used to cover American Pie at Shenfield Folk Club. We felt very cool and grown-up.

The chord progression is very strong and it's a terrific song to play.

Years later I met and interviewed Don McLean at Granada Television in Manchester, but to my disappointment he was not at all keen to discuss his biggest hit, and actually threatened to walk off set if I asked him anything about it. I've never understood what the problem was.

But that doesn't spoil memories of 1971, including a vivid mental picture of striding over a Welsh mountain on a warm summer night, heading back to an isolated youth hostel, singing American Pie with four mates at the top of our voices to the starry, starry night. Which leads me to McLean's other big hit, 'Vincent' – but that's another story.

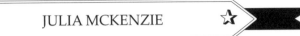

JULIA MCKENZIE

Actress and director

Broadway Baby

'Broadway Baby' from *Follies* by Stephen Sondheim. Singing this brought me in first contact with Stephen. I have rejoiced in his work ever since.

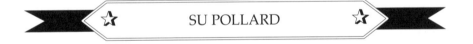

SU POLLARD

Actress

Happy Together by The Turtles

I have a very fond memory of a song by The Turtles, an American group who sang 'Happy Together'. I used to listen to it on Radio Caroline in the front room of our house with my boyfriend, Pete. It used to give me such a warm glow as it was 'our song' thinking it would be ours for ever. Unfortunately he left me for a girl guide!

Chef and TV presenter

Bye-Bye Blackbird by Nina Simone

It would have to be a classic track – 'Bye-Bye Blackbird' by Nina Simone, Live at the Village Gate. When my late mum listened to it she would do the sweetest soft shoe shuffle while cooking over the stove, and her arms became like wings flapping up and down to Nina's beautiful artistry on the keyboard. As Nina plays you out there is room to sing your own version of 'Bye-Bye Blackbird' to the end of the track which my mum did passionately every time.

My dad Chester, on the other hand, (a brilliant pianist himself and still alive) would just sit back, eyes closed, moving his head from side to side and pulling the most extraordinary facial expressions as the music and instruments changed, often smiling with joy and sweet memories. He saw her perform live many times. When I listen now I suppose I'm a combination of the two – which can sometimes be a little dangerous if I'm chopping onions.

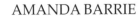

Actress

Looking for a Boy by George Gershwin

When I was about three I always used to sing this song. No matter where we went, my mother packed my music and I would perform it everywhere. Then, years later, I was starring in the Gershwin musical *Oh, Kay!* in the West End and the producer decided that he wanted to put another song into the show. When he asked me; 'Do you know "Looking for a boy"?' I exclaimed, 'I certainly do! But there's only one way that I can perform it and that's with the choreography my mother taught me to do when I was three!'

The producer told me to go ahead and do it just that way. When my mother came to see the show I didn't tell her I was performing it with the dance she had taught me as a child. When I did the number, I could hear her sobs from the audience!

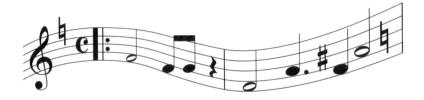

Comedienne

Lazy Bones by Paul Robeson

Hearing 'Lazy Bones' by Paul Robeson almost always transports me back to our family home in Kent. It's a Sunday morning, a summer morning because the windows are open and me and my brothers are out in the garden while Mum and Dad are peacefully perusing the papers and I know Mum will eventually get up and put the oven on from where eventually the cooking of Sunday lunch will blend with the smell of cut grass and that was Sunday. Lovely!

Paul Robeson was one of my dad's favourite singers, not only for his rich and gorgeous bass/baritone voice but for the impact he had on racial politics in America. Of course, that was all lost on me at the time but I so thank my dad for giving me the pleasure of knowing this hugely influential singer and through him a memory I will never forget.

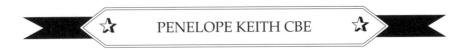

PENELOPE KEITH CBE

Actress

You Are My Sunshine

My earliest musical memory is of my late mother singing 'You are My Sunshine'.

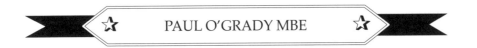

PAUL O'GRADY MBE

TV presenter, actor, author

I'll Take You Home Again, Kathleen

One of my favourite songs is a maudlin Irish ballad called 'I'll Take You Home Again, Kathleen'. My dad used to sing it when I was a boy and if I hear it now it still has the power to set me off.

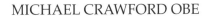
Actor and singer

For All We Know

'For all we know' is the song that evokes very touching memories for me. It was the tune that my mother and her first love would play every time he flew his Spitfire off into the unknown dangers, as part of the Battle of Britain in the Second World War. It was eventually a sad ending. He was shot down and died in early 1941.

SIR ALEX FERGUSON CBE

Manchester United football manager

Moon River by Johnny Mercer

My favourite song is 'Moon River' by Johnny Mercer. I just love the words to this song, they are fantastic, and in fact, it is my party piece!

Actress, scriptwriter and director

A Certain Smile by Johnny Mathis

'A Certain Smile' by Johnny Mathis is a song that never fails to stop me in my tracks and bring a tear to my eye. About twenty years ago, I was round at my mum's house and she and I were washing up when she confessed to me she'd had an affair with a young Polish immigrant called Craze back in the 1950s. I was shocked to see tears rolling down her face as I'd never seen my mother cry. She explained how they'd been lovers for a brief time until he'd been killed in a fairground fight. I was aware that her marriage to my dad hadn't been a happy one, in fact they divorced when I was three, but I had no idea that there was anyone else involved. My mother was not a glamorous or vain woman, she always put her children first. She was a hard-working and affectionate mother who never uttered the words 'men' and 'love' in the same breath. It became clear to me though, that she'd known deep, passionate love and had carried this man around in her heart for over thirty years and never been able to share the crushing agony of her loss with anyone.

She told me that 'A Certain Smile' was the song she and Craze had danced to when she first met him at a local dancehall. I wrote a play called A Passionate Woman, it premiered at the West Yorkshire Playhouse and went on to play for a year in the West End at the Comedy Theatre. Night after night I'd listen to that song and it never failed to move me to tears and more so now because Mum passed away four years ago. When I hear Johnny Mathis singing 'A Certain Smile' now it reminds me of my mum and I feel blessed that she met Craze and knew the love of a man and was, albeit fleetingly, truly happy.

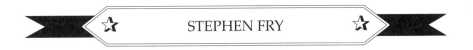

STEPHEN FRY

Actor, author, TV presenter

Love for Sale

I'm choosing 'Love for Sale'. It stirs up melancholy tinged with beauty and pity. A whole sad story told …

Novelist

Local Boy in Photograph by the Stereophonics

During the colder months of 2005 I spent a lot of time in my car driving between my home in Swiss Cottage and my mother's flat in East Barnet. I would arrive in the afternoons, after I'd finished work for the day, with my toddler Amelie strapped in the back and the radio on. My mother had been diagnosed with terminal lung cancer eighteen months earlier and had decided against another bout of chemotherapy, not prepared to fight it any more, happy just to let it happen. So for those few months I knew that every journey might be my last, that at any moment my mother might go from handing out biscuits and fruit pastels and having an opinion on the celebrity guests on the Richard and Judy Show, to being a dying person in a hospice, unable to chew or to care. Every evening as I left her apartment, my mother would come to her window and watch me and Amelie as we walked towards my car in the car park, and she would wave and smile.

'Wave,' I'd say to Amelie, 'wave at Nana.'

Then one afternoon her face did not appear at the window and I knew that we were entering a new phase.

I'd been stoic and philosophical about losing my mum. I

hadn't really cried. We are a family of pragmatists not drama queens. But that afternoon as my car headed home through the high streets of north London I turned on the radio and the song that was playing was 'Local Boy in Photograph' by the Stereophonics, a heartbreaking song about the death of a young man. I sang along and as I sang I sobbed, tears veiled my eyes. I blinked them away desperately, trying to keep my vision clear. And then suddenly, just as my eyes cleared, I approached a set of lights and a man landed with a thump against the bonnet of my car. I screamed.

'Oh my God! Oh my God!'

The man rolled off my bonnet and sprang lightly to his feet. He put a hand to his chest in a gesture of apology and continued across the road. As my car drew up alongside him on the other side of the traffic lights I rolled down my window.

'Are you OK?' I shouted across the road.

'Yeah,' he said, 'Yeah. I'm fine.'

And so I drove on, my hands shaking, the Stereophonics playing out the last bars of the melancholy song, my toddler asking me questions in the back, a man I'll never know walking home after a brush with death, my mother alone in her flat in Barnet, too ill to wave from her window at her eldest child and her youngest grandchild.

My mother died about three weeks later in May 2005, and still, whenever I drive that stretch of road, I hear that song in my head. I feel the sting of tears. I hear the thump of the man on my bonnet. I think about my mother. And whenever I hear that song, I am there in my car again, crying for my mother again, about to hit that man again. The whole thing is one big inextricable knot of feelings and emotions, the song, my mother, the man, the weather, very much like the lyrics to the song themselves.

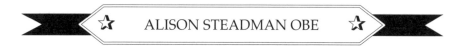

ALISON STEADMAN OBE

Actress

Rock Around the Clock by Bill Haley and the Comets

My sister's 21st birthday. I was 10 years old and very excited at her party. Her boyfriend (soon to be husband) arrived late and had fallen off the bus with Bill Haley's LP 'Rock Around the Clock' under his arm (my sister's present). He was upset that the record was damaged. We spent most of the evening dancing to 'Rock Around the Clock' and it always reminds me of that happy time.

My sister was married to him for fifty years when he sadly died three years ago.

He was a 'cool guy'.

Actress, TV presenter and author

Blue Moon

A song that always evokes fond memories and a smile is 'Blue Moon'. I can't remember the first time I sang it in public but it was my song of choice for every occasion especially when I'd had one too many.

As a girl I loved to learn all the old classic songs and would spend hours practising with a ping pong bat as a microphone. I could sing them all from Sinatra to Ella Fitzgerald. 'Blue Moon' became my standard and Mum and Dad would always make me sing it at family gatherings. If we were on long journeys I would happily bore everyone from the back seat of the car. All through my time at drama school I would bring it out at parties and clubs. It was my anthem. My mum was incredibly supportive of my theatrical aspirations even if she did not always agree with them or understand them. I miss her and my father so much and know they would have been so proud of me now. I will probably have to request that they play 'Blue Moon' at my funeral and I hope it makes everyone who knew me burst into laughter and not tears.

TV presenter, author, former wife of Rolling Stone Bill Wyman

Ain't No Mountain High Enough by Diana Ross

As a child I had a real love for music and when I was only four or five years old I remember my mum playing Elvis songs while doing the housework. I also play music now while doing my housework. (Thanks, Mum).

I choose the song, 'Ain't No Mountain High Enough' by Diana Ross because I used to hear the album advertised on the TV and I drove my family mad to buy it for me. I was eight or nine at the time and life was good. Christmas arrived and so did the album. I learned every song and every word.

At this time I lived on a housing estate in North London and my sister and I were lucky enough to live next door to two lovely Yugoslavian boys who became our best friends. The elder of the brothers was the local heart-throb and we were chuffed as he was 'our best friend'. After a few years of summer fun and much laughter he died at the age of 17 in a motorbike accident. It was such a shock, and seeing his little brother all alone was really painful. I hid my emotions from friends and family at the time, but I remember vividly lying on the floor next to a speaker playing my Diana Ross album listening to 'Ain't No Mountain High Enough' and I would sob my heart out – thinking of our friend whom we had lost. I now understand that was my way of grieving and I'm glad I did, as when I listen to the song now I smile and it brings back all the memories that we shared together as friends and neighbours.

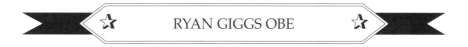

RYAN GIGGS OBE

Manchester United footballer

This is the One by The Stone Roses

'This is the One' by The Stone Roses. A great song that I never tire of hearing, as it reminds me of matchdays and running out onto the pitch at Old Trafford. It also reminds me of my childhood and growing up in Manchester.

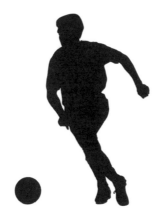

Novelist

You To Me Are Everything by The Real Thing

First, I need to tell you that I'm not Melissa. I'm her husband. Melissa died when she was 37 of breast cancer. Music was a very important part of her life and I think she would want me to contribute something on her behalf.

Melissa and I used to go dancing a lot. I remember the first time I saw her dance. She seemed to have positive energy pinging off her body. I loved dancing with her: usually we'd be whirling around the dance floor screaming along with the words, smiling, hugging, kissing.

The first time we danced to 'You To Me Are Everything' together, she looked into my eyes and held my face while she sang the words. It was like a thwack between the eyes for me – I realised that she really did think that I was everything to her – and suddenly I knew the depth of her feeling for me. And it made me cry – right there in The Mean Fiddler in Harlesden, with this wonderfully cheesy pop song playing. In fact it still makes me cry when I hear this song because it instantly fills me again with the love I knew she felt for me.

When someone dies I think we're left with the love we felt for them, but we lose the visceral, chest-expanding, brain-twisting feeling of their love for us. Being loved warms us, guides us, comforts us and motivates us. This song somehow reinstates that knowledge and that feeling.

In our later years together, this song came to mean so much more to us as we sang it to our beautiful baby – Sam. Our gorgeous boy arrived after Melissa's first encounter with cancer and we knew there was a chance that she'd have to go through it all again. In fact she had to deal with it four more times before this nasty, vicious disease sliced her out of our lives.

We would dance around the living room with Sam. He's seven now and he and I frequently sing it together while bouncing around the living room and thinking about his mummy – who he knows is living on a star and humming along with us. With a big grin on her face.

Andrew Saffron & Sam Nathan-Saffron

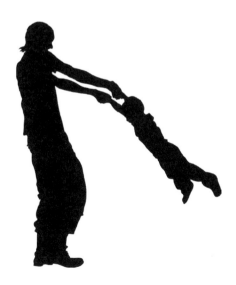

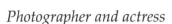

Photographer and actress

Teach Your Children by Crosby Stills and Nash

My happiest memory is with my daughter, free swimming with dolphins off the South Sea Island of Nuie. We wrote a piece about it for Harpers Bazaar.

It is a newish memory but the happiness of that time with her supersedes the many other memories that stretch further back in a long and eventful life. Tatiana sang to the dolphins underwater and they came right to her.

Author and former royal butler to Diana, Princess of Wales

My Heart Will Go On by Celine Dion

The song which invokes a strong memory for me is 'My Heart Will Go On' sung by Celine Dion as the soundtrack for the movie Titanic.

I have always been fascinated by the stories of ocean liners and particularly the tragic story of the SS *Titanic*. When it was built at the Harland and Wolf shipyards in Belfast in 1911, it was the largest man-made moving object ever built. It was a source of pride for the men and women who built her but it also mirrored the class system and social structure of that time.

The movie was released in 1997, which was a sad year for me. I have always told my children that every problem in life has a solution, except one … and when facing death we are always reminded of our own mortality, which we have no choice but to accept and move on.

The following year, I was appointed to the role of Fundraising Manager for the Diana Princess of Wales Memorial Fund and was invited to be a guest at a fundraising event during Oscar week in Hollywood. The event raised two million dollars for an Aids charity in Hollywood and the Memorial Fund. As part of the fundraiser, Asprey Garrard created a replica of the 'Heart of the Ocean',which Celine Dion wore at the Oscars to sing her song, the title track of the movie.

It was a bitter sweet night for me, a coalminer's son from Derbyshire meeting some of the most famous faces on the planet and remembering the one face who would have loved to have been there.

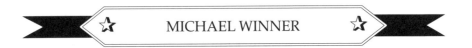

MICHAEL WINNER

Film director, producer and food critic

That's Amore by Dean Martin

I remember with great affection 'That's Amore' by Dean Martin somewhere around the mid 50s. To me Dean Martin had a better voice than Sinatra's and was the greatest all-round entertainer of the period, if not ever. I was such a fan of his that I used to take black and white film stills of Dean Martin to my tailor and say, 'Make a jacket exactly like this.' I then, with a stretch of imagination that beggars description, believed that I looked like Dean Martin!

SHARON GLESS

Actress

I Wonder What's Become of Sally

My father played the piano beautifully. As a little girl, I would sit next to him on the bench and sing along with him. He taught me all the words. Our favourite was an old song from the 1920s called 'I Wonder What's Become of Sally'. It was a sad song, but the way he sang it and the way he taught me to sing it – the phrasing and the pauses – I thought there was such beauty in the sadness. My parents divorced and my mother kept the piano, so I never heard him play it again. But I always remembered that song and how wonderful it was to be sad and thrilled sitting with my father on the piano bench. I ended up, many years later, sitting with him as he was dying, and I sang 'I Wonder What's Become of Sally' to him. He loved that I remembered.

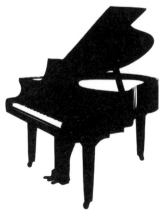

Actress, singer, author and former lead singer
with The Three Degrees

The Way We Were

Asking any singer to select their favourite song is always a dilemma as I have been in the business for quite a long time and have ever so many favourites. Songs come and go, the same as memories. From the first moment I heard Barbra Streisand sing this song, to the soulful version later recorded by Gladys Knight, to the production that is in my solo show, this song has always evoked a special place in my heart.

It always reminds me of how things used to be when times were good with The Three Degrees and just how different they can become when those times come to an end. The melody is as haunting as the memories. The lyrics are as poignant today as they were during the 1970s and the vocal deliveries from these great ladies of song make you feel the pain of loss.

It is therefore easy for me to see how the lyrics to 'The Way We Were' could be applied to the family of any Alzheimer's sufferer. When a family is torn apart, remembering the vibrant, intelligent person who has lost all control of their lives is frightening. So to those families, I send my very best wishes, prayers and the hope that in time science will conquer this dreaded disease.

Novelist

Teenage Kicks by The Undertones

I love everything by Punk band The Undertones, but I've chosen this track because it works for me on several different levels, mainly because it's forever linked to the DJ John Peel, on whose radio programme I first heard it in the late seventies.

So, it doesn't simply evoke one particular memory, one snapshot in time, but encompasses and defines a whole era of my life, from my teenage years right to the end of a long marriage, just as John Peel's constant presence as a well-loved voice on the radio did. If this means that playing 'Teenage Kicks' opens a Pandora's box of memories and emotions, the sour and the sweet escaping together, then so be it – and I wouldn't have it any other way.

Like a novel, a great song must contain the right mix of poignancy and joy to be truly wonderful and, for me, 'Teenage Kicks' has those elements – and right from the start, it's urgent and exciting In fact, I played it endlessly while writing my first romantic comedy novel, *Good Husband Material*, because the sexy voice of Feargal Sharkey inspired the main male character. I even gave him the same name, though in my head he didn't look remotely like Feargal Sharkey and definitely didn't play the same kind of music!

When I first heard the track in the late seventies, it was a time when I was struggling with many things – making a living while finding the space to paint and to write novels that were constantly rejected, trying (and repeatedly failing) to start a family … I'd like to be able to go back and tell that younger Trisha that soon she would be published, she would go on to have a wonderful son … and that her marriage would finally end, but it would turn out to be the best thing that ever happened to her.

But there again is the poignancy – when I heard of John Peel's tragically early death, there was only one person who had been beside me through all those years, to whom I wanted to turn to to share some of the shock and disbelief I was feeling – my newly ex-husband. And I couldn't: that door had closed.

It made me realise that to outlive all your close friends must feel much the same as divorce after a long marriage, knowing no one who shares your life-experience in quite the same way.

But 'Teenage Kicks' will always open the door and reveal all the riches and fool's gold of my life – and, in the end, it is a triumphant song.

Singer and philanthropist

Miss You Nights

I hope it's permitted to choose a song from my own repertoire! 'Miss You Nights' has always been one of my favourite songs but it never really held special memories for me until I sang it during my 50th anniversary 'Time Machine' tour in 2008. I performed it acapella, while projected on to a huge screen behind me were photographs of people I have known, loved and admired throughout my life, and who are now gone from us. From now on 'Miss You Nights' belongs to them.

I guess the choice of 'Miss You Nights' can also be related to those who have been taken from us by Alzheimer's (my own mother being one of them).

Actress

Je ne suis pas ce que l'on pense

From time to time, in totally different locations and circumstances, I find myself humming or singing quietly, 'Je ne suis pas ce que l'on pens-e… je ne suis pas ce que l'on dit'. It's the first line of a song my parents had on a 78rpm disc in my extreme youth – (the mid nineteen thirties).

I eventually learned the lyrics having been properly turned on to the French language at school, under a native French teacher, Henriette de Waligorski – I believe she had Polish antecedents – for whom I played Monsieur Jourdain in her school production of Molière's *Le Bourgeois Gentilhomme*.

'Melly', as she was privately known to her pupils, later took me to Paris where she had a flat, and introduced me to Bernard Frank, the son of her close friend, his mother. I fell in love with Bernard and seriously considered marrying him, (although it wasn't an actual affair, you didn't in those days).

However Bernard's speciality was Japanese demonology of the 11th century, and I found it hard to adjust to the idea of several years in Japan and the rest of my life in Paris, which I love as a city, but, still hoping to become a professional English actress, couldn't honestly consider as a permanent home.

Possibly as an indirect result of this early experience, my

English husband and I have a French daughter-in-law and three half-French grandchildren, and I still from time to time find myself singing quietly, 'Je ne suis pas ce que l'on pens-e' (I am not what one thinks).

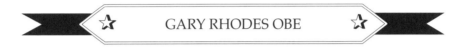

GARY RHODES OBE

TV personality, chef and restaurateur

Free by Stevie Wonder

A song that means so much to me is 'Free' by Stevie Wonder from his 'Characters' album. The song describes freedom for all and has such great life within it. On the off chance, I had the opportunity of seeing him perform this in the 80s and it has stayed with me ever since.

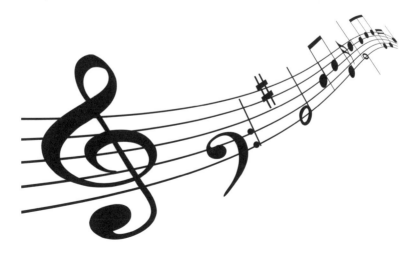

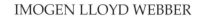

IMOGEN LLOYD WEBBER

Novelist

Glory Box by Portishead

Whenever I hear Portishead's 'Glory Box' it takes me right back to being a student at Cambridge and spending long evenings listening to the blaring jukebox in Girton College's bar. It was the song of the moment and evokes a very specific time in my life.

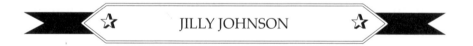

JILLY JOHNSON

Model, singer and author

Isn't She Lovely by Stevie Wonder

The moment I hear Stevie Wonder singing 'Isn't She Lovely' I get goosebumps and a warm rush of nostalgia engulfs me, for it was in the same summer of 1975 when Stevie warbled those lyrics, that my daughter Lucy was born – and yes she was lovely!

Actor, singer

Beautiful Saviour

I certainly relate to your efforts on behalf of Alzheimer's as my mother is presently suffering from the mean cruelties of this disease … as did my grandmother. June (my mum), who just turned 90, has been afflicted for the past 10 years and is now in the final stages. She knows no one and, of course, can't speak or look after herself. She and my father, who died three years ago, were married for 64 years and after he passed, she kind of gave up. "Where's Dick?" she used to say, "I haven't seen him for such a long time." He used to dress her and put on her earrings and lipstick in the mornings.

Now, bless her, she's in great physical shape, but is essentially gone. She's being cared for at an Alzheimer's Unit at Golden Empire in Grass Valley, California and, thankfully, my sister Lois and her husband Richard are near by to look after her. Needless to say, it's been a gruelling few years for them and as well, for us five siblings as we watch this vibrant, genius of a woman dissolve. The only thing that is still alive is her brilliant blue eyes and the one thing her eyes respond to now is music. She was a very fine contralto/mezzo soprano who sang the 'Lieder' (the songs) of Shubert and Shumann and Brahms and, in her college days, she used to sing in one of America's foremost college choirs. Her favourite hymn was 'Beautiful Savior'. She was also a teacher of English and German … a lecturer … a soloist with the local symphony and a brilliant organizer.

We spent nearly six years in Berlin after the war (1949 to 1956), as part of the reconstruction period, where my dad … a history/political science professor and pastor, served refugees, those escapees from eastern Europe … putting members of families who had fled into Berlin back together with their families who had escaped to the West. One of the beautiful gifts given to us as a family by these folks who had virtually nothing were the German rounds and the Bach cantatas that we learned.

Over the years my four brothers and sisters and our children have carried on the tradition that was begun with my mother. When we visited her this past Christmas at Golden Empire (the Alzheimer's unit in Grass Valley) and sang the rounds for her, her eyes showed that she recognized 'something'. Then, we sang 'Beautiful Saviour' and she smiled in that sort of twisted, uncontrolled way that she does now and moaned her response. Still, it was recognition and she took my hand and squeezed it. You are so right about music being one of the few connections that we can make with the afflicted. How wonderful … even for one moment. Music is the key.

Actress

The Sky Boat Song

My mother sang it to me as a lullaby when I was a baby and saw it made my bottom lip tremble.

I sang it to all my children when they were tiny and watched their lips tremble too, a primal response to something that touched them deeply, something between melancholy and joy.

Now I sing my grandchildren to sleep and see their mouths tremble as that same song penetrates their small beings, something ancient, something to do with the change from major to minor.

The song? 'The Sky Boat Song'. And as my dear old Ma danced down the Dementia Road I would, years on, sing it to her, returning the favour. And it never failed to bring sharp brightness to her eyes and cause her lips, not to tremble but to chuckle upwards into a smile of pure delight.

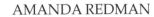

AMANDA REDMAN

Actress

For Emily – Wherever I May Find Her by Simon & Garfunkel

I have many favourite songs but I think the one I'd like to pick is Simon & Garfunkel's; 'For Emily – Wherever I May Find Her'. I first heard it when I was fourteen and fell in love with the tune and lyrics. I vowed then that if I ever had a little girl, I would name her Emily, which I did. Even though the song is not about a baby, the lyrics in the last couple of verses describe exactly how I felt when Emily was born.

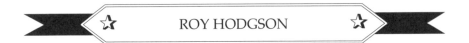

ROY HODGSON

West Bromwich Albion football manager

Sonny Boy by Al Jolson

The song is 'Sonny Boy' by Al Jolson. There are so many songs I would have liked to choose as I like many different forms of music and there are so many songs I have fallen in love with over the years.

The reason for choosing this Jolson classic is that it reminds me of my ludicrous impersonations designed to impress my future wife, and takes me back to a time when being light-hearted and 'devil may care' was the norm rather than the exception.

NEIL SEDAKA

Singer, pianist and songwriter

It's All in the Game by Tommy Edwards

In 1958, my wife and I just started going steady. 'It's All In the Game' by Tommy Edwards was an enormous hit. We would find ourselves making out with it. It became our song because of its wonderful emotion and sentiment. Being a songwriter, the hardest thing to do is write a simple piece. This does the trick.

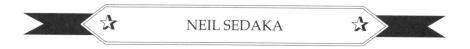

Actress and author

When I Fall in Love by Nat King Cole

I think music more than anything else can evoke a memory, a moment or an emotion, and it can send you travelling back in time to the place where you first heard it, or the person you heard it with. It can produce a vivid recollection of something special, either happy or sad.

I have many musical reminders of things, some connected with my children or grandchildren, or friends, some that make me laugh or want to cry, but perhaps the one that has always brought back happy thoughts and happy times is Nat King Cole singing 'When I Fall in Love'.

The very first time I heard it was with Bryan. We were celebrating our first wedding anniversary. We were in Los Angeles and we'd been invited to hear Nat King Cole in concert. We were given ringside seats and I gather someone had told him it was a special night for us because not only did he dedicate 'When I Fall in Love' to us, but he sang it to me. It was one of those fabulous moments you never forget. So I'm sure you'll understand why Bryan and I have always regarded it as 'our song'. Whenever I hear it today I am reminded of that occasion and memories come flooding back of the many happy times we've spent together since.

Singer/songwriter and actress

Angel Eyes

'Angel Eyes' is a song that's very special to me. My mom, dad and several of my five brothers had great voices. The boys had a singing quartet which I wasn't allowed to be a part of because not only was I too young, but I was a girl! My mom used to sing around the house all the time, and I greatly admired her voice. A short time after having had surgery on a goitre she was trying to sing and found she couldn't hit the notes. She turned to me and said, 'Sing that for me baby, will you?' Well, you would have thought it was a command performance for the Queen of England! I didn't even know that she knew I could sing. I was so thrilled I nearly couldn't sing! The song was 'Angel Eyes'.

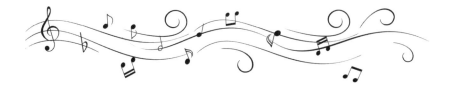

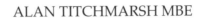

TV presenter, novelist, gardener

Groovy Kind of Love

'Groovy Kind of Love' is the song that reminds me of my first proper girlfriend when I was 15. Hearing it now still generates those butterflies in my stomach!

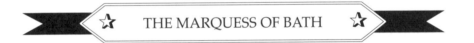
THE MARQUESS OF BATH

The Last Time I Saw Paris

My special song would be 'The Last Time I Saw Paris'. This is the first ever pop song that I remember learning by heart.

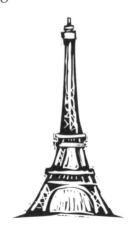

Singer

What's the Matter Baby by Timi Yuro

The song 'What's the Matter Baby', written by Clyde Otis and Joy Johnson for the late Timi Yuro, who has to be one of the greatest singers who was around in the 60s, always gives me goosebumps.

In 1988 I did an album called 'Bookbinder's Kid'. On that album I did a tribute to Timi and sang 'What's the Matter Baby'.

That year I did a tour to promote the album. Having come off stage one night and enjoying a drink with my family in our motor home, Timi called me on my new mobile phone (quite a thing then) to tell me she thought I did a fantastic version of the song.

What a woman she was! She could hardly speak then because of the cancer in her throat, but she just wanted to make contact.

I have to say it is one of the proudest moments in my career.

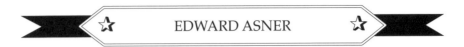

EDWARD ASNER

Actor

Cat in the Cradle by Harry Chapin

My choice is 'Cat in the Cradle' by Harry Chapin.

The song simply and powerfully evokes the sadness of not being an appropriate parent.

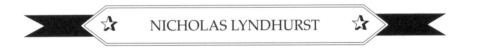

NICHOLAS LYNDHURST

Actor

Afterglow by Genesis

I have many favourite songs, but I think perhaps one of my best loved must be 'Afterglow' by Genesis, from an album called 'Seconds Out'.

Author

The Man I Love by Billie Holiday

Can music spark off memories other than our own? That's what I think when I listen to Billie Holiday's beautiful tones, so redolent of melancholy. Because one bar of 'The Man I Love' and I'm me and her simultaneously, in the Deep South with the shimmering sun rising outside a smoky club and yet somehow, also at my desk in cool, crisp Wicklow.

The music lays down a hypnotic beat that makes me fall into that other place, like muscle memory helps people play the violin and evolutionary memory helps the finger-sized baby kangaroo instinctively crawl up its mother's belly to the safety of her pouch. Music crosses all barriers of time and place, cradling us in warmth.

For the last ten years of his life, my father had dementia and the parts of him that were the last to go were his memories of the far past. Yesterday was gone from him but he talked of 'going home', when home was a big red-bricked house miles away from our home, the one he'd lived in for thirty years.

He loved music, from the classical tapes he collected the old LPs of jazzman, Bix Beiderbecke. As a family, we feared the words dementia and Alzheimer's as terrifying bogeymen. It was as if those words themselves had power and, until we got a diagnosis, the words could not be real. But they were.

In those years, we thought the right thing to do was to keep his dementia from him. We were mute when he yelled that all the paintings had been moved, and why were we doing this to him?

Now, I wonder if music could have helped? If listening to the music he loved could really have soothed the savage breast? In a world that must have seemed like a surreal painting, the soft murmuring of jazz or classical music might have brought him quickly to a happier time.

I'd do it differently now. With the benefit of hindsight, I think he should have known the truth. But we were only trying to help, to soothe as best we could.

We never listened to Billie Holiday together. He loved jazz before I did and he liked different sorts. Louis Armstrong's gravelly 'Mack The Knife' was one of the few we both adored.

But when I hear Vivaldi, I can still see the cover of the tape he loved of 'The Four Seasons'. I can see his desk with all his tapes and papers neatly organised, along with his fountain pens. There might be a bit of paper out, filled with his tiny, obsessively neat handwriting in the dark blue ink he favoured.

'The Four Seasons' brings me back. Like magic. But then, music is magic.

Actress and author

Hymn to Freedom by Oscar Peterson

Music is vitally important to me. My father was a musician, traditional jazz and popular dance, and I grew up in the company of musicians. I would sit for hours in empty auditoriums listening to the bands rehearsing. At our olive farm in the south of France I have over 3,000 CDs and on my ipod almost two years worth of music. Making choices is therefore always difficult and quite impossible to pick one piece but if I must I am going to say Oscar Peterson's rendition of his own composition and now a jazz classic, 'Hymn To Freedom'. I don't know how many albums of his I have with this stirring piece on it and, for me, even the pauses are full of soul and yearning. Duende. My husband Michel used to put this on every morning as he brought me my coffee in bed and I was woken to this rousing and spirited tune. What an inspiring way to begin any day. We saw Oscar's last concert in Paris and by mistake he played 'Hymn to Freedom' twice and I could not have been more delighted. He was barely able to shuffle onto the stage and had to be led by two men, one on each arm, but when he sat down at that stool and lifted his hands to the keys, it was as though a muse entered him. His body language changed entirely. He was upright, strong, lost within his interpretation of the music. The audience was spellbound. Oscar Peterson, one of the greatest of twentieth-century jazz musicians and composers. RIP, Oscar. I hope they supplied him with a piano when he stepped through those Pearly Gates.

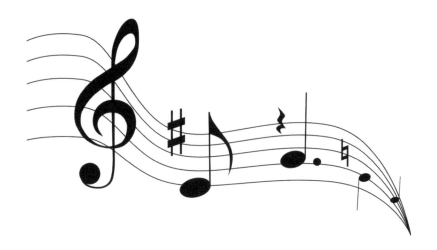

BILL ODDIE OBE

Author/actor/tv presenter/musician/conservationist/artist

Nothing Compares to You by Prince

I was a 'war baby'.The first song I heard was probably something on the wireless . Maybe 'We'll meet Again' by Vera Lynn, or perhaps Gracie Fields' 'Sally'. 'Our Gracie' and I were both from Rochdale. The first song I sang in public was 'Christopher Robin is saying his prayers'. A traumatically embarassing duet with a little girl at a school concert. We were both six years old. We had to stand on a table, hold hands, gaze into each other's eyes and deliver such lines as 'God bless nanny, I think that's right. Wasn't it fun in the bath tonight!' Ah the austerities of the post-war years. Mixed bathing in a tin tub!

I met my first wife, Jean, in 1963, when she was 'headlining' at the Establishment Club in Soho. She was a singer, with a great voice and a fabulous repertoire. If I had to resuscitate musical memories of her, I'd say just about anything by Rogers and Hart. Jean and I are no longer married, but we are still good friends, and much of our contact has a musical content. Records, concerts, and particularly singer songwriters. The same shared enthusiasm applies also to my second (and current) wife Laura. She would be thrilled to be associated with all kinds of showstoppers from musical film and theatre. Top of the list: the whole score from *Little Shop of Horrors* which we saw in New York, in a ramshackle little theatre, off off Broadway, before it became a movie and a worldwide hit.

What neither I, nor Jean, nor Laura, nor any other romantically associated lady, have ever had is what couples commonly refer to as "our song". Writing this piece has made me realize that I don't generally experience music in terms of recalled emotions and memories. I know this sounds a bit literal – or maybe a little pompous – but I don't treasure a song because it reminds me of some event or other. I revere it simply because it is a great song and/or a great performance. The music IS the memory. If I have to choose one song to persuade the doubters, or simply to induce my own goosebumps, it is 'Nothing Compares to You' (or '2 U', in Prince text). A lot of people probably think of it as a Sinead O'Connor song. She did a great version, but she didn't write it. Prince did, and – to misquote Carly Simon – nobody sings it better, as I have had the spine-tingling pleasure of experiencing several times over the years. On most of those occasions, I have felt very emotional – a lump in the throat, a tear in the eye – not because I am remembering a lost love, or reliving a heartache, but because I am privileged to be hearing a great singer songwriter doing what they do – making music. If I am sharing that experience with an equally enraptured audience, so much the better. Whatever your taste, there is no denying the power and the joy of music. They can't take that away from any of us.

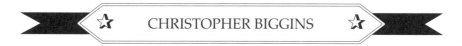

CHRISTOPHER BIGGINS

Actor

What Do You Get When You Fall in Love

My very first love affair had its ups and downs. I'd been to see a new musical in the West End called *Promises, Promises*. There was a song called, 'What do you get when you fall in love' and during the downs I used to play it and cry my eyes out.

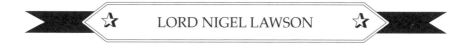

LORD NIGEL LAWSON

Politician and author

London Pride by Noel Coward

Noel Coward's wonderfully sentimental and patriotic song 'London Pride', which dates back to 1940 or 1941, brings powerfully back to me memories of the war years, when I was a schoolboy living sometimes in London and sometimes in the country.

Broadcaster and journalist

Look for the Silver Lining

At home, we all sang anything we liked. It was the soundtrack of my childhood, sometimes funny, sometimes rude, sometimes obviously important if only to the singer.

My mother (born 1900) had a small true voice and she always went back to a song, the refrain of which was

"A heart full of joy and gladness

Will always banish sorrow and strife

So always look for the silver lining

And try to find the sunny side of life"

Silver linings weren't soppy maunderings for people who had lived through two world wars.

And the refrain would come back to me whenever things were rough.

Then, five years ago, in the television showing of a documentary on American musical theatre – torn between tears of recognition and desperately looking for a pencil to write it down – I heard Marilyn Miller (born 1898) singing the song my mother sang for us.

I've heard it all these years as if she sang it to me.

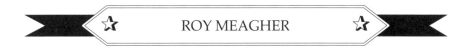

ROY MEAGHER

Actor

Simply the Best by Tina Turner

I hate dancing, but Tina Turner's 'Simply the Best' almost makes me get up and have a go.

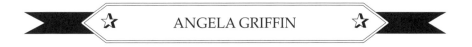

ANGELA GRIFFIN

Actress and TV presenter

You're All I Need to Get By by Marvin Gaye
and Tammi Terrell

My most memorable song is 'You're All I Need to Get by' sung by Marvin Gaye and Tammy Terrell.

We actually had my best friend Nicola Stephenson read the lyrics of this song at our wedding at Babington House in 2006. It pretty much summed up how we felt. It makes for a great karaoke song too with the husband after a couple of wines!

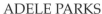
Novelist

Life's playlist:

A song that instantly makes me want to dance

Groove is in the Heart by Deee Lite

I love dancing; I'll dance to anything that is likely to be played at a wedding reception, if you know what I mean! 'Groove is in the Heart' is a winner. I love the way it starts, "We're going to dance, we're going to dance. And have some fun." It's irresistible; it demands lots of arm waving and hip shaking! I ought to confess that my enthusiasm for dancing way out strips my expertise!

A song I'd choose to sing at Karaoke

Hey Big Spender by Shirley Bassey

My rendition has been perfected over 30 years. I've adored the tigress from Tiger Bay since I was a tiny girl. She's all about gusto, passion, zeal and ambition. Plus this song can be belted out without too much attention being placed upon pitch (a serious advantage for me!)

A song that always cheers me up

Let Me Entertain You by Robbie Williams

I love Robbie Williams. I think he's an astounding entertainer, a phenomenal talent; arguably a bit too big to fit comfortably into this world. I love many of his earlier tracks but 'Let Me Entertain You' is particular fun; it's wry, brash, and boisterous. It reminds me of a brilliant day and night I spent at his Knebworth gig a few years back. An experience that was so overwhelming I've incorporated it into my latest novel, Love Lies.

A song that reminds me of being a teenager

Should I Stay or Should I Go by The Clash

I was a teenager in the 80s and had little interest in the popular music of the time. But, every Friday, from aged 15 to18, I religiously pitched up at the local nightclub, 'The Kirk' where non-pop, surprisingly cool tracks were played. It was there I discovered Nina Simone, the B-52s and many others. I dated a broody, unbelievably cool boy, called David, and we used to dance to this track at the Kirk. We never smiled at each other when we danced but we never broke eye contact; it was sooooooooo sexy. Of course, because of our age we had an on/off relationship and because of our age we were quintessentially self-focused; I think we both seriously believed this thrashing, edgy song spoke to us alone, that it was written about our breakneck dash through romance. Just for us!

A song that reminds me of heartbreak

Never Ever by All Saints

Whenever a woman is ditched she goes insane with wondering what she did wrong while in the relationship and why it ended. This track perfectly sums up that bleak mystification, shock and vulnerability. It's simply heartbreaking. If only we spent as long on listing what was wrong with him and why we were better being rid of him!

A song that always makes me cry

Come What May by Ewan McGregor and Nicole Kidman

As featured in the glorious film *Moulin Rouge*. The words to this song are so utterly romantic, in the biggest sense of the word; dreamy, impractical, passionate and noble. It's a love song about unconditional love; it always makes me think of my husband and my son, as I used to sing this to my son as a lullaby when he was a baby. I like to play it on full blast and boo with happiness that they are in my life; this song makes me feel so damned grateful. Seriously, go and listen to the words, think about the people you love, and I bet you'll boo too!

Novelist

Judy Teen by Cockney Rebel

One of my favourite songs is 'Judy Teen' by Cockney Rebel. It doesn't seem to be played that often on the radio now, but hearing the sliding synth as it starts still makes the hairs on the back of my neck stand up.

I was about thirteen when my friend, Andrea, and I were given tickets to see their show at the Stadium in Liverpool. My friend's older sister had a boyfriend who was a ticket tout and we thought that was a fabulously glamorous job, even though we had no idea what it actually entailed. All that we were concerned about was the steady supply of free tickets that came our way for great concerts that none of our peers had a hope of attending. We were the envy of our classmates. Together we saw The Jackson Five, The Osmonds, The Temptations and many other iconic bands of the time. But the Cockney Rebel concert was special – it was the first time we were allowed to go to Liverpool on our own on the bus. I remember we took hours to get our outfits together. We scoured charity shops until we had our own bowler hats like Steve Harley did and we duly decorated them with glitter. Our faces were also daubed with glitter and inexpertly applied eye liner. In black T-shirts and tight jeans we thought we looked the bees knees. We sat on the top of the bus all the way to Liverpool, singing 'Judy Teen' at the top of our voices. The concert was wonderful and we sang until we lost our voices.

I practised and practised what I thought was a marvellous dance routine employing a broom handle as my cane and singing 'Judy Teen' became my 'turn' at family gatherings. Thank goodness there was no video then.

Not long later, I was in America on holiday with my parents when Andrea phoned to say that Cockney Rebel had announced their split. We cried transatlantic tears of grief. How would we replace the hole in our lives? Well, fortunately, Roxy Music came along very soon after and our fickle teenage hearts were given away once more.

But whenever, I hear that song, I'm back on that bus with Andrea. In fact, I might just go and play it now. Pass me that broom handle!

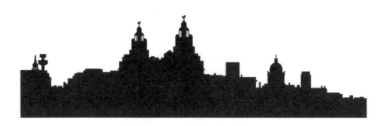

Actress

Maria from Bahia by Chuy Reyes

When I was about 14 years old my father rented a seaside cottage next to my grandparents house in Sweden.

One night I watched my mom and dad dance to a song that has never left my head, 'Maria from Bahia' by Chuy Reyes. It was a Grammofone and it was a very special evening for me as my parents didn't usually display such romantic behaviour, and I can still see them dancing and I never forget the song!

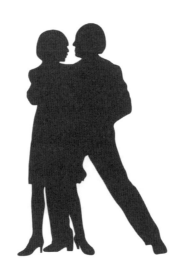

Author

Entry of the Gladiators by Julius Fucik

My favourite piece of music is 'Entry of the Gladiators' by Julius Fucik. This unbelievably jolly tune always heralds the start of circuses – and as my dad was a circus clown it was his theme tune. And I remember my mum and dad prancing about to it in our kitchen when I was a child and everyone laughing. It's a stirring, foot-tapping, unforgettable piece of music – and now it always makes me cry a mixture of sad and happy tears. Nothing on earth reminds me so much of my dad or those wonderful childhood days when my parents were alive and I innocently (and luckily!) thought we were all immortal and had no idea of the heartbreak the future would hold. 'Entry of the Gladiators' was played at the start of my dad's funeral (at his request!) and everyone was tapping their feet and weeping buckets at the same time. So, even though it makes me cry every time I hear it, I still love it because it brings my mum and dad and my blissfully happy childhood back to me for just a little while.

Media personality and author

Almost any record by Eartha Kitt brings my childhood flooding back. Through her I began to understand the power of sex appeal as her curvaceous frame and unabashed vocal come-hithers inspired the lust, worship and awe of any red-blooded male, very much including my father.

Eartha ('A man has always wanted to lay me down but never wanted to pick me up') began to purr and prowl her way through myriad now-legendary songs in the 1950s, when Orson Welles famously proclaimed her 'the most exciting woman alive'.

Always described in every feline term imaginable, the illegitimate child of a black Cherokee sharecropper mother raped by a white plantation owner, I was totally fascinated by her and remain so to this day, nearly 25 years after her death.

'Santa Baby', 'Just an Old Fashioned Girl', 'Uska Dara', 'C'est si bon' – the list of her hits is endless. Her records were constantly played at home and I will never forget the evening, when I was about 12, and my parents and a group of friends came back from seeing her live at the Winter Gardens in Bournemouth. They were all, ladies included, glowing with the excitement and thrill of her performance. If you don't know who and what I'm talking about, I urge you to seek her out now. I'm off to play 'My Heart Belongs to Daddy.'

Novelist

Time in a Bottle by Jim Croce

Jim Croce wrote this song in 1972 and dedicated it to his unborn son, Adrian. Less than a year later, the talented songwriter lost his life in a plane crash. He was thirty years old.

'Time in a Bottle' became a huge hit posthumously as did many of Croce's songs. Luckily for the world he left behind, he had completed his last album just eight days before the crash and so left a further legacy of beautiful music for us to enjoy.

I was only a child when this poignant evocative song with its haunting melody became a number one hit. My big brother had bought the album (that's like a CD for those of you too young to remember) and I played it every chance I could. I remember liking all the songs but there was something special about 'Time in a Bottle' in particular and I immediately fell in love with it.

Perhaps it was Croce's untimely death – young, emotional girls are suckers for sad endings. Perhaps it was because I was on the brink of puberty and drawn to songs of romance and love and you can't get more romantic than,

'I'd save every day like a treasure and then,

Again, I would spend them with you'

Perhaps it was the beautiful guitar music that, literally,

seemed to pluck at the heart strings or the simple, but striking lyrics that would touch the hardest heart. Or maybe it was a combination of all of the above.

Now, all these years later, when I listen to the song, it's from a different perspective. I hear it as a parent and there are lines that have me reaching for the tissues

So this is the song I choose; this is the song that evokes memories of a happy, carefree childhood and reminds me today how important it is to live each day as if it were the last.

'Time in a Bottle' moved me all those years ago. How wonderful it is to discover that it still has the power to move me today.

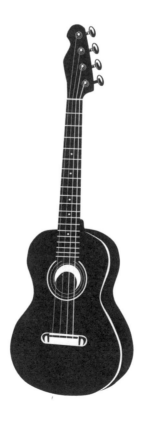

Novelist

The Glass Mountain by Nino Rota

My brother and I were put in orphanages when our mother died, but in 1951 when I was six, and Michael eight, our father married again and we were brought home again to find we had a new sister, nine-year-old Selina, later to be adopted by my parents. Hilda, my stepmother, had a wind-up record player, and a stack of records. 78s in those days and Selina and I played them all the time. One record in particular stands out: 'The Glass Mountain' by Nino Rota. We would put on a couple of gauzy nightdresses that Hilda had put in our dressing-up box, and dance. Selina was graceful and good at dancing, I was like a carthorse, but the beauty of that music made us both think we were good enough for The Royal Ballet, and we would play it over and over again until the needle wore out.

Sometimes we included Michael, our brother, in it, but then we had to make it into a play. Michael was always a Prince, Selina the Princess, and I was mostly the Witch. It was me who had the ideas for the plays, but no words were ever written down, I told the other two what they had to say.

I heard 'The Glass Mountain' again just the other day, and I was taken back to the early 50s, there in that nightie, rouge on my cheeks, an artificial flower in my hair, dancing joyfully with my new sister. Life wasn't terribly good with my stepmother, but we three children could escape into fantasy each time we put the record on.

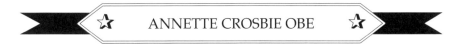

ANNETTE CROSBIE OBE

Actress

Simon Smith and His Amazing Dancing Bear
by the Alan Price Set

What immediately comes to mind is 'Simon Smith and His Amazing Dancing Bear' sung by the Alan Price Set because it's the song I used to sing to my children when they were both too young to understand it. It was a great tune to hold them in my arms and dance to. Forty years later, they still remember the words.

Novelist

Smoke Gets in Your Eyes by Brian Ferry

The song I'd choose would be 'Smoke Gets in Your Eyes', sung by Bryan Ferry.

I must have been about fifteen when Bryan Ferry released an album of cover versions of classic songs. I was a dippy teenager who had just discovered boys. I was flooded with dreams of romance and love, all I could think about was the object of my affections. This would change frequently – a boy who'd looked in my direction at the bus stop, the man who ran the dodgems at the fair, my second cousin Martin who was in his 20s and had a red sports car. All were completely oblivious of me, which was fine as I think I would have been horrified if there'd been any sign of reciprocated interest. As far as I was concerned there was nothing as satisfying as wallowing in the miseries of unrequited love.

Bryan Ferry was another unobtainable hero. He lounged across the album sleeve in a white tuxedo, jet black hair drooping over one ice blue eye, a languid hand holding a cigarette. He was sophisticated, suave, cool and impossibly attractive, just the sort of man who would never look at a gauche, plump teenager like me. But in my dreams ... I would watch the vinyl disc spin round and drift off into a semi-hypnotic state where I could wear a bias-cut white satin dress and live in the South of France drinking champagne and eating wild strawberries. My hair would be sleek instead of curly, my hip bones would jut out instead of being smothered in layers of puppy fat, my fingernails would be long and scarlet instead of bitten and stubby. I would smoke and drink cocktails and a man like Bryan Ferry would fall madly in love with me.

All the tracks on the album were wonderful but my favourite was 'Smoke Gets in Your Eyes'. It spoke of passionate love and inner suffering, both emotions I strongly identified with, and romance – which I yearned for. I would play the record and weep along with Bryan, full of regret and sadness for lost relationships which had never existed. My mum spoilt it a bit when she claimed to know all the songs. How could she?! She was old and knew NOTHING AT ALL about true love, about which I, of course, was an expert. And then, at the school disco, Phil Thompson kissed me, and I left Bryan for the real world.

But just thinking about the song brings back memories of that dreamy, summer hovering on the edge of growing up, leaving behind the child's world, looking forward to the adult world but not quite ready to move on. 'Smoke Gets in Your Eyes' sums up those self-indulgent months, full of romantic fantasies and laced with yearning, sitting alone in my bedroom with tears streaming down my face and perfectly happy.

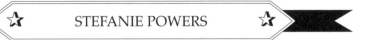

Actress

Thanks for the Memory by Bob Hope

As most people who are a part of the baby boomer generation will remember, 'Thanks for the Memory' was the signature song of Bob Hope, whose weekly appearances on television were an institution for every American family. Mr Hope, who was my neighbour in Palm Springs California, had countless versions of the lyrics to that song including X-rated ones. But the song became much more of a personal experience when I was doing my very first one-woman show which was a musical retrospective of my life with visual projections on a screen. Singing 'Thanks for the Memory' to a montage of photos of William Holden was a special moment that will always make me feel an intimate attachment to that lovely song.

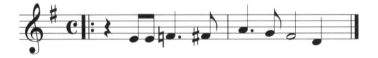

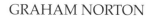

GRAHAM NORTON

Actor, TV presenter and comedian

Chain Reaction by Diana Ross

Diana Ross singing 'Chain Reaction' brings me back to youthful wild nights out in London town. I once gave myself a black eye in my rush to get on the dance floor when I heard it.

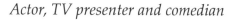

ESTHER RANZEN CBE

TV presenter and journalist

From May to September

'From May to September' was my late husband Desmond Wilcox's favourite song. It was sung at our wedding (our second to each other, the first was a civil ceremony in a Register Office) and Dame Cleo Laine sang it at his memorial service. I find hearing it intensely moving.

Comedian

Feelings

I have had experience of a loved one with dementia, my aunt Rosemary had it. I have since built a six-bedroom wing on St Clare's Hospice in Newcastle On Tyne.

Rosemary who was dying of cancer was also developing dementia. I visited her in hospital. She was taking off her dressing gown as I passed her room and I started to sing 'The Stripper' amid hilarious laughter from patients and staff watching her doing The Stripper as I sang. Then I told the family a joke about Michaelangelo who went to the doctor with a pain in his neck and back.

The doctor looked at him and said; 'Ceilings you must stop painting ceilings'.

So that is my song, 'Feelings' I always think about Rosemary when I hear that song. We had a photograph taken together which she had enlarged and I put on it 'To Rosemary from your secret Irish Lover' and the staff were telling me every time someone went into her room she would say; "This is my boyfriend Frank Carson, He's a cracker!"

The last time I saw Rosemary was seven weeks later at her funeral. Every time I hear the song 'Feelings' I say a silent prayer for Rosemary.

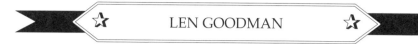

LEN GOODMAN

TV star and professional ballroom dancer

Your Feet's Too Big by Fats Waller

I have lots of songs that mean a lot, however, when judging *Strictly Come Dancing* I see trouble with footwork. A track jumps into my head from Fats Waller whose style and personality just make you feel good. The track: 'Your Feet's Too Big'.

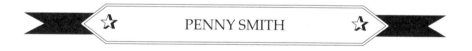

PENNY SMITH

TV presenter and author

Crazy

My choice would be 'Crazy'. I did a duet show on BBC with Curtis Stigers. On the first night, I was seriously rubbish. I blame it on the fact that you can hear yourself back through the speakers. So I decided to do 'Crazy' in the style of Marge Simpson from *The Simpsons*. We were voted back in! And it's such a great song.

SUE MOORCROFT

Novelist

My Simple Heart by The Three Degrees

My dad, Walter Moorcroft, loved to sing along to the radio and was well known in the family for getting lyrics wrong. But I thought he'd surpassed himself when he said, 'What's that pimple song?'

'Pimple song?' My memory didn't easily supply a song about a pimple.

'It's on the radio all the time – "My Pimple Hurts".'

He sang it for me. I fell about when I realised it was 'My Simple Heart', by the Three Degrees. Whenever I hear that song, I think of Dad. And I listen closely. Actually … it does sounds as if they're singing. 'My pimple hurts'.

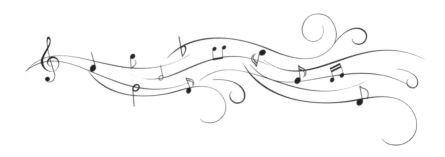

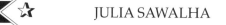

JULIA SAWALHA

Actress

It's a Wild World by Cat Stevens

My father used to speak the lyrics to me as I would leave for work or a night out. Whenever I hear it, I feel a deep, overwhelming love for my father.

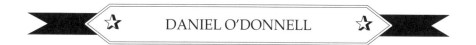

DANIEL O'DONNELL

Singer

I Just Wanna Dance With You by Daniel O'Donnell

The song I'm going to choose is one I've recorded. Like many of my generation *Top of the Pops* was the highlight of the week on TV. I watched it without fail. I never thought I would get to appear on it. In 1992 I recorded a song called 'I Just Wanna Dance with You'. It became a hit and I was on *Top of the Pops*. Every time I sing or hear the song it reminds me of that event in my life.

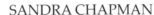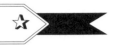
Journalist and columnist

Prologue / Crunchy Granola Suite by Neil Diamond

A night in 1973, seven months pregnant and my unborn child was restless. Perhaps he was sensitive to my nervous state.

Each night his father was dodging the bombs and bullets in downtown Belfast where he worked as a newspaper sub-editor. His route home was through one of the worst areas of the city. Worrying about him had become a nightly ritual.

I'd tried pacing the floor. Going to bed wasn't an option especially with the kicking I was getting. It was late and I was too anxious to tackle any domestic chores. Then I remembered that earlier that day I had bought an LP. Would music calm my nerves? The LP was 'Hot August Night' by Neil Diamond. I had heard about this amazing album and put it on the record player. I was more of a Rolling Stones fan but didn't think 'Jumping Jack Flash' would have had much of a soothing effect on my nervous state.

I sat down on the settee and tried to get comfortable as tiny feet pummelled away. I couldn't hear much from the record player, just musical notes. Then they got louder and I heard what sounded like classical music. Had I bought the wrong LP?

The music got louder, the notes higher. This was leading

to a crescendo of some kind, notes hanging in mid air, I was enthralled. And then came the beat, crashing into my senses, enveloping me in a kind of wonder. The two of us in fact. I realised my little one had heard it too because he'd stopped thrashing around and by the time the first few tracks were over he was either alseep or desperately waiting to hear what was going to come next.

The first track in this album is the famous 'Prologue' leading seamlessly into 'Crunchy Granola Suite'. This was pop music as I'd never heard it before and from that night I became a lifelong fan of Neil Diamond.

I've never forgotten those two particular tracks. Whenever I hear them I'm transported right back to that night of mixed emotions, the joy of knowing I was going to have a baby, with the anguish of not knowing if his father was going to survive to see him born.

In fact his father got home safely at 4 a.m. It had been a particularly bad night of trouble and he had literally been driving through gunfire on the streets.

His nerves weren't up to much either so I insisted he listened to this amazing music starting with the Prologue. He loved it too and all three of us slept well that night.

Next day, when he went to get into the car for work, he found two bullet holes on the rear door of the car. Much later he told me he knew the car had been hit but just kept driving. In fact he had been driving my car that night, a much longer, heavier and more sturdy model than his own. I don't like to think what might have happened had he taken his own car that night.

Novelist

Go or Go Ahead by Rufus Wainwright

I don't have an all-time favourite, but certainly there are songs that evoke particular times in my life. I love Rufus Wainwright's 'Go or Go Ahead'. When I was coming to the end of my marriage I was living on a very old farm in the country, and I would drive along the country lanes in an old pick-up truck with this song blaring out of the stereo – it made me feel that anything was possible, that only good things lay ahead. I still can't hear it without feeling that same swell of optimism and hope.

Novelist

La Vie en Rose by Edith Piaf

When I was little, I loved my Nana's big black musical box with the Chinese drawings on the outside and on the inside the bright red velvet lining and the mirror and the little ballerina who would twirl to the music that began as soon as the lid was opened. The tune, although I didn't recognise it at the time, was 'La Vie en Rose'. My nana was an avid reader of love stories and my granddad was a rough-edged Barnsley miner and part-time wrestler with a poet's soul who loved the arts. It was he who told me all about the meaning of the song – how love makes you see the world through a bloom of lovely pink – and 'The Little Sparrow' who made it her own. They had a lovely home, immaculately clean, big cosy chairs, a lit fire and a kitchen where baking was always taking place. In and out of the house would wander their Chow dog – Granddad always had Chows – and whenever I hear 'La Vie en Rose' I am back with them, eating home made bread and butter still warm from the oven, the Chow at my feet looking at me wistfully to share. And Nana bustling around with a duster, Granddad humming along to opera, telling me the stories behind the music. 'La Vie en Rose' brings tears to my eyes every single time I hear it– sad ones that they are no longer alive to see that I became a writer (and bought a Chow), and sweet ones because I have such warm and wonderful memories of them to treasure. Their essence has become one with that tune.

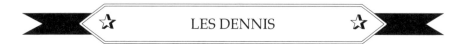

LES DENNIS

Comedian, TV presenter and actor

In My Life by The Beatles

Whenever I go home to Liverpool I find myself singing 'In My Life' by The Beatles. I went to the same school, Quarry Bank, as John Lennon so "the places I remember" that he sings about are also the places that evoke memories for me. It seems to be the primary song in the soundtrack to my life.

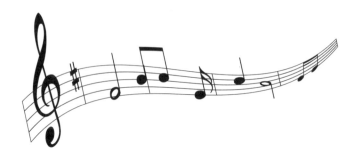

Singer, actress and TV personality

To Sir with Love

A song that has a very special place in my heart is 'To Sir with Love'. When I was only 16, I was given the opportunity of a lifetime – to act in a movie alongside the legendary Sidney Poitier. As if that wasn't daunting enough, I had the task of recording the title song for the film … I am so proud to have been involved in this piece of film history and to have helped bring this song to life.

To create the title song, I worked alongside a songwriter called Mark London. I had to cajole him to take the time to write a melody that would work for my voice – but when it did happen, it all came together in one afternoon. We then contacted the renowned lyricist Don Black, who has written such classics as 'Born Free', 'Diamonds Are Forever', 'Man with a Golden Gun' – and 'To Sir with Love' came to life.

Being associated with this no.1 classic hit is amazing – but the memories it conjures up for me are more personal. I was a very naïve teenager who didn't realise until many years later how significant the movie and its themes were. This was a film that could not have been made in America at the time. It would have been utterly socially unacceptable for white people to have any kind of a relationship with a black person or have any physical contact at all. It was a successful film with audiences world-wide – but it seems to have earned a special place in the hearts of the American audience because of its political significance at that time. People often approach me to tell me touching stories of how much this groundbreaking film meant to them and how much it has resonated throughout their lives.

At Sidney Poitier's 76th birthday, Oprah Winfrey talked about how Sidney had paved the way for her – and for many black people - in life. I am so proud to have worked with Sidney and that *To Sir with Love*, our work, is a part of history.

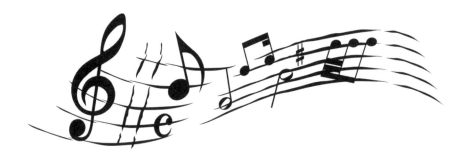

Actor

Clair de Lune by Claude Debussy

I have many songs which hold a special place in my soul from my earliest memories to the present day. Music has always been foremost in my life, for my Welsh mother loved singing and my Irish father was a musician (piano, accordion, tenor sax, clarinet) and a dance band leader. I played guitar and drums in several groups in the sixties. My mum and dad's song was 'J'attendrai' and I still treasure a copy by Django Reinhardt and Stephane Grappelli … sadly, I no longer have a wind-up 78 rpm gramophone! My favourite song of all time is 'Hound Dog' by a young man called Elvis Presley. It is my animal song and continues to send jive pulses to my old legs. However, my poetic interior prefers 'Clair de Lune' by Claude Debussy. This was used in a little film I directed called *Flower Children* in which my first born starred as an unborn and baby. It was also played at my father's funeral.

Novelist

I Don't Like Mondays by The Boomtown Rats

1979. It happened when I was in my third year of secondary school. A Thursday evening, just after tea, and I was across the road at my friend Alison's house comparing homeworks. Top of the Pops was on, her little brothers squabbled and cursed under the bay window, her mother was sorting through a basket of washing and her dad sat in the corner smoking his pipe. So far so normal.

Suddenly, from the TV, came the most tremendous glissando and then four thumping grand piano chords. It felt like the overture to something really important. I couldn't help but look up, and there on the screen was Bob Geldof, sneering at me. He was breathtaking. Never had I seen anyone so simultaneously ugly and gorgeous.

By the time I'd caught up with what the lyrics were about – a school shooting incident – the scene had changed to a living room uncannily similar to the one I was in with its floral sofa and Queen Anne style coffee table. And look, the dad was in his shirt sleeves like Alison's father, and the mother doing housework too. Then a beautiful young schoolgirl, of whom I was instantly jealous, walked in and sat down sulkily next to Bob. He became wilder and angrier, his hair sticking up more and more as the dramatic tension mounted. I don't know what aspect of the song bothered me so much – the crashing piano arrangement, the fact that the video featured children like me, the macabre subject matter or Bob's lips – but I was skewered. As Johnny Fingers pounded out those last gloomy bars, I knew something inside me had changed for ever.

Because up to that point I'd been an old-fashioned, bookish child, overweight and awkward, scornful of teen pop culture because it frightened the pants off me. My favourite pastimes had been cataloguing fungus and copying out Tennyson poems. The only single I'd bought to date was a non-threatening folk song called Clog Dance by Violinski and even then I'd got my mother to go into the scary record shop and buy it for me.

Back home and desperate to record the Rats track, I spent the next few days surfing stations on my transistor radio. The trouble was, DJs then had all been primed to talk over the intro or final bars of every song they played as a deterrent to the 70s equivalent of illegal downloaders. Home Taping was Killing Music. This meant it was near impossible to capture a complete track without some clunking false start or abrupt cut off. Finally I gave up, caught the bus into Bolton and braved the HMV in the precinct to buy the album.

'I Don't Like Mondays' had tipped me out of childhood. I started listening to John Peel's late night show, drawing anarchy signs on my school exercise books, alarming my mother by singing Dead Kennedys lyrics. Two years later I'd passed through punk and was a heavy metal fan, painting Hawkwind logos on the back of my denim jacket. I'd slimmed down, learned how to use make-up and become a bit of a liability all round.

Had I understood that evening, with the Rats chanting in my face and Alison's brothers scrapping on the carpet next to me, that these changes were on their way, I'd have flat-out panicked. But I didn't have a choice. Like the girl in their song, something had got switched inside my head and I walked out of that house a different girl from the one who'd trotted up the path, her homework under her arm.

Adolescence beckoned and it was going to be a bumpy ride. There was no going back; Bob had spoken.

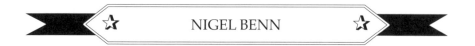

NIGEL BENN

Professional boxing champion

In the Air Tonight by Phil Collins

My song is 'In the Air Tonight' by Phil Collins, as it is the song I came out to in my second fight with Chris Eubank.

Politician and TV star

One of Those Days in England by Roy Harper

This song, from the early 1970s, evokes for me the long hot summer of 1976, the simplicity of life at home, and the essence of what English folk music is all about. The lyrics really depict an idyllic atmosphere, all that is nostalgic, popular, and potentially lost from today's world. Every time I hear the song, I recall those gentle emotions. It was a long time ago when the song was written, and even longer since England really was like that. But occasionally, as I drive through the back roads of the land, I'll see a speckled village green, a thatched roof or traditional old pub, and find myself humming this song.

TV presenter/actress (and former Blue Peter presenter)

You Are My Sunshine

My mother always sang. She had a wide repertoire: snatches of music hall ditties, carols, songs from the shows, Noel Coward tunes, old favourites with new lyrics ('Hark the Herald Angels Sing, Mrs Simpson stole our king'). She sang while she cooked, or cleaned and always at our bathtime. My sister and I can't remember a time when we didn't know every verse of 'O Little Town of Bethlehem', or when we couldn't sing all the way through the 'Gloria' in 'Ding Dong Merrily on High' without gasping for breath. Forties and Fifties songs were popular too. And then, one day, making our way through 'You Are My Sunshine', I suddenly added a harmony. Only a simple one – a third above, but nevertheless enormously satisfying. Who sang the song before? Who cared? We owned it! We could have sold tickets! It became our tune, always thrilling and true. We've sung it to our children and now that she isn't with us, we sing it in our mother's memory .Like her love, like our childhood, for me that song is as warm as a cuddly towel after a hot bath.

Singer/songwriter/musician

A Rainy Night in Georgia

Putting aside my angst-ridden teenage years when song titles changed as frequently as each lost love, I have chosen 'A Rainy Night in Georgia' written by Tony Joe White. I sang this song after buying Brook Benton's version produced by Arif Mardin, who was also producing my album in 1972. By 1982, the song was a highlight of my repertoire. I was a fully fledged troubadour, one man and his guitar, singing 4–5 hours a night in strange foreign places, travelling alone, where, because of various languages spoken, conversations were limited to 'Do you support Manchester United?'. There were many of us troubadours scattered like lost souls in places like the Arctic Circle, and Northern Europe where the landscape was snow and ice and the days invariably dark and dreary. The accommodation was equally grim and dispiriting.

We all had similar stories to tell but after a few years I grew to like the life in bars. Whenever I see James Stewart in the film *Harvey* I am reminded of the countless colourful and amusing characters I met in those places and of his unique approach to life . 'No one ever brings anything small into a bar' he says in the movie. How true that was. (These days, the critics attribute that line to Tom Waits!).

I spent many hours thinking alone of loves lost and of the terrific highs I'd had in London during those magical optimistic gloriously happy years of 1967-8-9. I knew I would be unlikely to find someone willing to put up with such an insecure lifestyle, no matter how colourful it became. I was a drifter in a Western movie, or a double-agent in a John le Carré spy story, or a gambler in Vegas or Havana. The lyrics of the song tell the tale of a guy on his own, drifting from place to place. It helped me; to adopt a role to get through it all. Sometimes I felt nuts enough to even wish I was a spy as the wages would have been better and I would have known how to defend myself. I had nearly 20 years of that strange life and managed to get through the loneliness and despair, clinging to my dreams and believing in them.

By 2001 when 'How Wonderful You Are' became a big hit, I had already become established locally in the south of England and regularly played at The Talking Heads in Southampton. It was that song in that place that caught the attention of my present and for ever love of my life. After Sue had doggedly spent months and months slowly de-thawing my frozen emotions of 20 Arctic years, we finally reached that state of 'and they lived happy ever after'.

I still sing the song occasionally for it was that song that accompanied me along the long journey that led to the amazing life I have now.

Novelist

Your Feet's Too Big by Fats Waller

Actually this tune summons up TWO memories, both intensely happy. It's Fats Waller's 'Your Feet's Too Big'. Anything by Fats, of course, fills one with joy; my first memory is of my father introducing me to Fats' music, by playing me this record when I was around eleven. If you don't know it, it's about the singer's girlfriend who is perfect in every way except for her enormous feet. Many years later I fell in love with Mel Calman, the cartoonist, another Fats fan, and also an admirer of my vast feet (size 8). Mel was not only smaller than me but had niftier little feet. He always liked tall women and with that comes, of course, nice big feet. In fact he used to draw jokes about them; I remember one drawing of my foot which was folded like an accordion, which when opened out practically stretched across the room. The lovely thing is that both the song, and the two men in question, were filled with enormous affection about the subject. I'm sure they all understood that large feet are preferable to small; they keep you upright better.

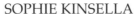

SOPHIE KINSELLA

Novelist

Short People by Randy Newman.

I first heard it in the Holywell Music Room at Oxford. It was sung by an undergraduate I vaguely knew called Henry Wickham – and when I heard him sing I immediately thought, 'He's got to be mine'. I pursued him quite shamelessly and now we've been married 19 years and have four children! Whenever I hear 'Short People' I'm transported back to that moment.

JOAN COLLINS OBE

Actress and author

The Way You Look Tonight

My favourite song is 'The Way You Look Tonight'. We played it for our first dance at my wedding to Percy Gibson.

Novelist

She by Charles Aznavour

I must have been about four years old and I was sitting in the front of my mum's convertible Morris Minor. You could back then. It was the 70s and no one was interested in seat-belt laws and child seats. It was all flower-power and free love and flares the size of sailing masts.

It was a hot, sunny day and we were driving home from the school with the roof down, listening to the radio. And suddenly this song started playing, 'She' by Charles Aznavour, and Mum started singing along.

I'd never heard it before and didn't know any of the words, but I'll never forget that moment. Never forget listening to the song and looking across at my beautiful mum, with her long brown hair and the teeniest of mini-skirts, and thinking he must have written the song about her. It was a moment of complete happiness and love.

I'm forty now, and my mum's seventy-one. But now, whenever I hear the song, I'm right back there again; a little four-year-old girl next to my mum, in a bright yellow Morris Minor covered in flower stickers, with the top down and the sun on our faces. And now I know all the words and sing along.

TV presenter (and former Blue Peter presenter)

You're Still the One by Shania Twain

When my husband and I got married in 2000, a very good director friend of mine, Penny Ewing, who I met when we both worked on *Blue Peter*, shot a film of our wedding which is so beautiful that to this day I cannot watch it without crying. It really was an amazing day and she captured the emotion and mood not only through the lens but by the use of music and knowing all of us so well. She presented me with the film using Shania Twain's 'You're Still The One' as the main sound track and I really do consider it now "our tune" and every time I hear it, it evokes beautiful memories of a wonderful day.

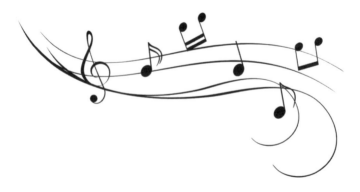

GORDON RAMSAY OBE

Chef, TV personality and restaurateur

Yellow by Coldplay

'Yellow' by Coldplay brings me back to when our flagship restaurant was awarded its third Michelin star. I used to listen to it on the way to and from the restaurant and I'll forever associate it with that feeling of pure elation when I found out.

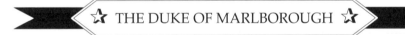

THE DUKE OF MARLBOROUGH

On the Sunny Side of the Street

I have always very much liked 'On The Sunny Side of the Street', with lyrics by Dorothy Fields and music by Jimmy McHugh. This song has been sung by many well-known artists, and as I have always been called "Sunny", I have always enjoyed listening, and sometimes dancing, to this lively tune, which helps one forget the problems that exist in the world today.

Journalist and author

Heartbreak Hotel by Elvis Presley

It happened in 1958 or 1959 (I can't quite remember which) and I was about 12. I was walking from the bus stop to the flats where we lived, an estate called The Green, in Liverpool 13. It was late afternoon in summer and I had been to visit a friend. We had been playing my precious Elvis Presley LP, which I now clutched proudly under my arm as I dashed home for my tea. My favourite song was the melancholy 'Heartbreak Hotel' and I was singing it in my head when suddenly I heard running footsteps behind me.

I'd just reached the patch of grass on the left, where the estate began. In the distance I could even see the edge of our living room balcony. A violent shove sent me sprawling and my LP was torn from my grasp. About five boys, aged around 13, encircled me, jeering and egging each other on to insult me.

'Who'd want to kiss 'er – she's ugly!' crowed one.

'Show us your knickers'.

'She got no tits'

And so on.

I was an innocent, skinny, plain, bespectacled girl, who

(unlike some of my friends) had never experienced even those childhood flirtations which can cause such unhappiness. Most of the time I lived 'down at the end of a lonely street' in my head, never feeling I belonged in any world except the ones within my bookshelves. Now the ugliness of what I was hearing terrified me. I watched them pass my record from hand to hand. Elvis smiled his snarly, lop-sided grin from the flame-coloured sleeve. I wanted my dad to come racing down and scatter them with his fists, but he couldn't see me any more than Elvis could. There was nobody around to help me.

'Let's steal 'er record' somebody said.

It was only then that I began to cry.

You always hope that in any group there will be one person with a conscience, for whom cruelty is not the default setting. Someone who will feel a bit of pity. Maybe realising that then was the foundation of my innate optimism. For I heard one say, 'Aw, la' – give 'er the record'.

Maybe they wouldn't have listened to him, but then came the warning, 'Somebody's coming'.

So my LP came spinning down, striking me painfully on the arm, as the gang whirled away and ran back the way they had come. Ahead, two nurses were strolling along the path from Broadgreen Hospital where, in 1946, I was born. In those days nurses wore starched white caps and aprons. No wonder they looked like angels to me. They stopped by the weeping child, bent down and asked. 'What's the matter, love?'

'Nothing,' I sniffed, scrambling up and clutching Elvis to my heaving chest.

I ran home and told my parents nothing at all. Even then I knew you have to be brave – always. But ever since that day the song 'Heartbreak Hotel' reminds me of the time when I realised that, no matter how loved you are, no matter what you achieve in life, no matter how many joys light your way, your soul will always be on its own. That's how it is. And that Heartbreak Hotel is a real place, 'always crowded' indeed.

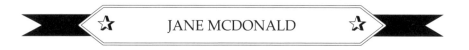

JANE MCDONALD

Singer and TV presenter

I Love You Because by Jim Reeves

I thought I would tell you about a song that reminds me so much of my father who sadly passed away in September 1993. My father and I used to go ballroom dancing twice a week to our local Working Mens' Club, just an organist and drummer and a glass of pop, but my father was a lovely dancer and a great teacher. His favourite dance was the foxtrot and the song that always makes me smile and think of him is 'I love you most of all because you're you' by Jim Reeves.

Fashion designer

Rock the Boat by The Hues Corporation

The summer of 1974 was a very confusing year for me, I was 19 and finding out who I really was, what I wanted, and where I wanted to be. Learning to accept the man I was meant to be.

During one very hot summer morning with no classes that day, I decided to pull on my favourite cut-off shorts, beat-up sneakers and high school T-shirt and got into my trusty little Toyota and headed for the ferry leading to a special place – The Pines on Fire Island about 20 minutes from where I grew up. Having heard so many stories about the glamour and the people, I set off with butterflies in my tummy to this exciting new place. Just to put you in the real mood it was the days of Calvin, Bianca, Halston, Andy, the whole Studio 54 set. As I approached the island I heard music emanating and it was 'Rock the Boat'.

It seemed so fitting during a time of ambivalence to hear those corny but poignant lyrics. I remember loving the volume, the bounce, the sheer high octane disco beat. I was jumping out of my skin. I felt I belonged finally.

That day as the crowd danced barefoot, sun-kissed and carefree, a person who looked to have just jumped off a Marlboro poster came up to me and said, "Listen you have everything in front of you, remember, brown eyes are soulful, blue eyes are beautiful, but your green eyes are the best. I can tell from looking at you you're going to go far – real far kid!'

Me, the skinny, lanky, green-eyed boy, was full of smiles that day!

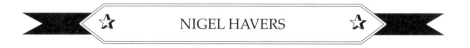

NIGEL HAVERS

Actor

No Reply by The Beatles

I used to be in a band called 'Crinkle' in the late 60s, early 70s with my brother and a couple of other friends. The only time I was allowed to be lead singer was while the others were taking a break, and this was my song. I still love it!

Radio presenter

Raining in My Heart by Buddy Holly.

I guess this song would usually be a memory for most men regarding an ex girlfriend. For me it will always be a reminder of one of the closest and dearest friends of my wife Marianne and myself, Simon, who was tragically killed in a road accident in 1993. He was just 38 years old and he died because of somebody else's stupidity. Simon was the most helpful and loyal friend to all who knew him which is why it was so hard to come to terms with, that song keeps him close to us always. Music has been a major part of my life since I was a child and as it has the power to make us laugh or cry I don't believe it will ever be surpassed by any other method of affecting our innermost feelings.

Author

All That She Wants (Is Another Baby) by Ace of Base

I was giving birth to my daughter in Barnsley General Hospital. It was 1993, and that summer's hit single was by Ace of Base, and it was called 'All That She Wants (Is Another Baby)'. I didn't like it much, but it was tremendously catchy, and it was playing in the little room in which I was in labour for 24 hours. It still brings back that time; the bilious pastel-coloured walls; the chemical smell; my husband trying to spritz me with a water spray and getting his head bitten off for his pains, and, through it all, that song with its thumping, moronic bass line playing on the radio for what seemed like the thousandth time – and trust me, the LAST thing I wanted right then was the prospect of another baby. All my plans for a natural birth, the whalesong, the herbal teas, the Bach flower remedies – poof! Out of the window. All I wanted right then was for them to get the damn thing out of me. And then the sun rose, and she was there, and her eyes were the blue of the Earth as seen from a great height ...

Journalist

La Femme d'Argent by Air

On November 12th 2000 I gave birth to my first baby. I remember waking up at dawn with a tremendous feeling of peace and yet anticipation. I stood up and my waters broke in flood, thrillingly, as I stood, stone still at the end of the bed. My husband was sure the birth would 'take days' and talked me back to bed where I lay wide-eyed and exhilarated for two whole hours! The first contractions passed, ebbing and flowing ever more strongly, until at 9 a.m. we arrived at the Royal Free in London. Getting undressed in the room where I would finally see our much longed for child, I kept saying 'put the song on put it on please put the song on!' in between puffing until my husband put on that tune that would play on a loop for the next four hours. It is by the French group Air and is called 'La Femme D'Argent'. It took me away to an amazing place, I remember shouting at Craig at one point, 'The beach, the waves can you see the waves can you see them?'

And then there was this sticky, warm, perfect little girl child lying across me, nuzzling for her first drink. And I will never, ever forget that song as long as I live.

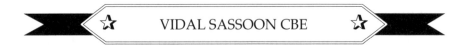

SAMANTHA CAMERON

Wife of the Prime Minister of the UK

The Snowman

The song that I would love to choose is 'The Snowman'. It reminds me of Christmas with the children as they have been to see it at the theatre a few times and adore it. They listen to it every Christmas and it is a song that the whole family love.

VIDAL SASSOON CBE

Iconic hairdresser and businessman

Everything I Have is Yours by Billy Eckstine

I grew up with Billy Eckstine, he was my favourite and there was one very special song I played almost on a daily basis. It was called 'Everything I Have is Yours,' but as a fourteen-year-old shampoo boy I had nothing to give, except a great desire to improve the lives of my family, which I was eventually fortunate enough to do. I'm playing him now as I write this little note to you.

TV presenter, author and model.

Blackbird by Paul McCartney

My song is 'Blackbird' by Paul McCartney. It was 1975 and I had just married David Bailey, we were in Hawaii visiting my family. I was in love, but upset that my parents had divorced that year, and my mom was now seeing a younger man. Paul and Linda McCartney had come to Hawaii with their children, Stella and Mary, who I would sometimes babysit. I thought Paul and Linda the most perfect couple in the world and I wanted my marriage to be just like theirs. Paul was very sweet to me and helped me to understand my mother better. I have never forgotten that kindness. This song always reminds me of him and his lovely family. My parents went through a couple of marriages each, but then decided to remarry nearly thirty years later. When Mom passed away in 2007, she was happily married to my father.

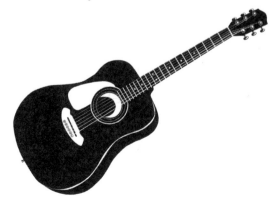

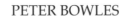

PETER BOWLES

Actor

You May Not Be an Angel (because angels are so few).

It was 1951, I was aged fourteen or fifteen and it was the first time I had worn long trousers. I waited for my new girlfriend to come and meet me. I sang the above song to keep myself warm in the freezing weather. She never turned up.

I later discovered she was out with my best friend!

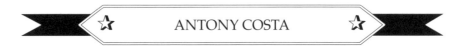

ANTONY COSTA

Singer, songwriter and actor

I've Got You Under My Skin

The song 'I've Got You Under My Skin' reminds me of when I was a young lad and my mum used to sing it. She said it was my granddad's favourite song. He used to sing it when he was in the army. It's a very beautiful song.

Actress/ author /Polish Countess

Calling All Angels by Kiki Dee

One of my favourite songs which holds many memories happy and sad is Kiki Dee singing 'Calling All Angels' from her album 'Almost Naked', I first heard it close to the time after my mother died and since then it has resonated with me through moments of sadness and loneliness, but always with faith and trust. 'Calling all angels…. Walk me through this one…. Don't leave me alone.' A kind of a hopeful call to the powers that be for spiritual guidance and protection. In fact it is a song I would love to have played at my funeral.

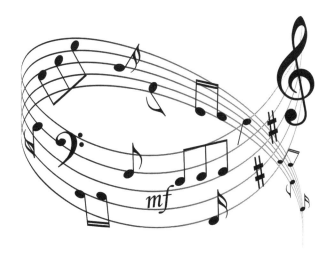

TV presenter and actor (former Blue Peter presenter)

Alright, OK, You Win by Joe Williams

I could pick many pieces of music that evoke memories, but the one I have chosen is unusual in that it is from the first concert I ever saw, and I have been totally hooked on Big Band Swing ever since. I saw Count Basie and His Orchestra at The Grand Theatre in Blackpool at Easter 1954. It was a memorable event for me, as I was at boarding school and we didn't get out much. The one most memorable thing was, it was the first time I had really watched a singer just stand at the microphone and sing. He was the legendary Joe Williams, and he came on and sang six numbers and brought the house down. He was fantastic! One of the pieces was 'Alright, OK, You Win'. And it blew me away. I was in New York in 1976 and in a small music bar in Greenwich Village one night, my wife and I wandered in, just by chance, to find that Joe Williams was performing. He sang with a small five-piece outfit and his voice was as lush and as beautiful as ever. I just had to speak to him, and after the gig I managed to introduce myself, and reminded him of the Blackpool concert on that 1954 tour. He remembered it well, and was thrilled to meet me, and to tell me that he married a Blackpool girl, and spent quite a lot of time in the UK. I've never been a great one for fan worship, but Joe Williams was, and is, to me, one of the greats, and that number evokes some of my happiest musical memories.

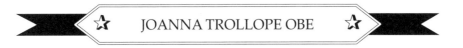

JOANNA TROLLOPE OBE

Novelist

La Mer by Charles Trenet

My father suffered from vascular dementia for well over a decade before his death, and, towards the end, had a long period of not speaking in English, but instead, in the atrociously accented, grammatically impeccable French he had learned as a young man before the Second World War. So for him I'd choose Charles Trenet singing 'La Mer'.

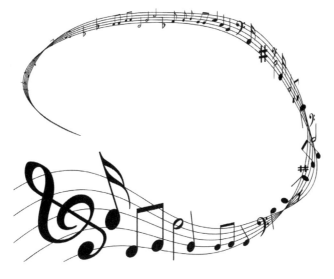

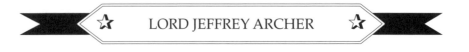

LORD JEFFREY ARCHER

Novelist and former politician

If I Never Sing Another Song by Joe Longthorne

One of my favourite songs is 'If I Never Sing Another Song' by Joe Longthorne. It reminds me of Joe's amazing ability to fight back against cancer.

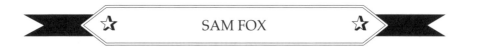

SAM FOX

Singer, actress and former glamour model

The Miracle of Love by Annie Lennox

'The Miracle Of Love' by the fantastic Annie Lennox always brings back an amazing memory of 12 years ago when I met my current partner, Myra. At that time I was at a bit of a low point in my life. Then one night, we were snuggled on the couch and Myra played 'Miracle Of Love'. It sent shivers down my spine as the words were so apt, she told me she loved me and I told her she was a 'Miracle Of Love!!'

Impresario

Please Please Me by The Beatles

A tune that never fails to evoke a happy feeling is from a time in my life that was a watershed: The Beatles – 'Please Please Me'

The Beatles record was a number 1 hit and I had just booked them for £65 to appear at the Black Cat Club in my local church hall, but because of demand we moved to the Azena Ballroom. I negotiated from the local telephone box with Brian Epstein and we haggled for two days until we agreed on £65. This was a huge amount of money in those days. I met the boys at their hotel and brought them to the Azena – it was a tremendously successful night and lots of fun.

They were a great bunch of kids going through their first taste of success and, of course, destined for stardom and I thought, I want some of that, and from there my success continued also.

So every time I hear this tune the hairs on the back of my neck stand up and the whole feeling of that night comes flooding back.

Writer, TV presenter and creator of The Rocky Horror Show

Tutti Frutti by Little Richard

We read that Saint Paul had a special moment while on the road to Damascus. When we undergo a moment of revelation, it is very often described as a Damascene moment or, a Pauline experience. Mine, although not quite as spiritual, is as follows: it was 1955, I was a thirteen-year-old boy strolling along the Strand in Tauranga, a 'then' small town in New Zealand's Bay Of Plenty. I was passing a milk bar called, believe it or not, The Candy Store. A girl I knew slightly was working there and she called me in off the street. 'Hey, Richard,' she said, 'listen to this.' She flipped a coin into the slot of the jukebox that stood on the shop floor. The jukebox lights pulsed, the motor whirred, the machine picked up a side-loaded disc and dropped it onto the turntable, the arm swung across, the gritty sound of the needle as it hit the groove hissed out through the speakers and then: Oh Lord! Hot Damn! I heard Little Richard screaming- "AH WOP BOP A LOO BOP A WOP BAM BOOM. TUTTI FRUTTI ALL ROOTY". And his voice stabbed me like a long shard of broken glass. A high priest of rock and roll had called out to the faithful and I was enslaved.

Author, journalist and showbiz reporter for 'This Morning'

The Flumps theme

Well I've gone for the Flumps theme tune. As played on Grandfather Flump's flumpet. Everyone else probably opted for opera classics and Ivor Novello winners in this book and looks really learned, but, you know, Pootle, Perkins and Posie have got me through a lot in this life.

You know some days you just wake up and you're just cross? You're just grumpy. Some days, no matter what anyone says to you, no matter what anyone does, there's a black cloud over your head that just won't shift.

On days like this – have a Google if you can. (Bear with me on this, I promise it will work) Put in The Flumps and The Cloud – and find the episode when Perkins the Flump gets into a bad mood when a grey cloud gets stuck over his head.

'It's a too much morning,' Perkins sighs as his Flumpy friends try to blow away the gloom-causing cloud to no avail. 'I feel ...umpty. I'm a fed-up Flump.'

That's just how you feel some days. Sometimes you just can't see the nice side of a morning because you're under a cloud.

I send the episode link to any friend having a bad day. I defy anyone, even the umptiest of Flumps not to watch the episode and at least raise a slightly grumpy half smile of recognition.

Perkin's cloud. It goes in the end of course. Black clouds always do, eventually. Laughter and friendship chase them away and the grey times go.

But just a couple of notes of the theme tune are enough to lift any cloud-laden days for me. It raises a smile and stops me being such a fed-up Flump. And for that, it's my favourite tune.

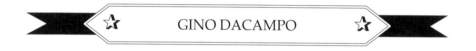

TV chef

Don't Look Back in Anger by Oasis

My favourite song is 'Don't Look Back in Anger' by Oasis. The song reminds me of my arrival to the UK in the 90s when Oasis were the rockband of the time. It is my motto for life, as life is too short!'

YASMIN ALIBHAI-BROWN

Journalist and author

My mother Jena was often beaten down by fate but she always came back up again, fighting, laughing, covering up her fears and sadness that settled into her early on, when she was seventeen and locked into a marriage to an older man, my father, brainy and bold, but not a husband who understood what his wife and children needed. In her last years as she got more frail, she was able to recall her life more vividly and honestly than ever before. We always had on wistful, melancholic old Hindi songs while I cooked her favourite dishes and made notes, recorded precious memories later published in my memoir *The Settler's Cookbook*. The songs were about betrayal, disappointment, heartless societies and careless men. We cried and she talked, an exile's stories awakened by music and stirred by food too. I listen to them now every evening as I cook and often cry too, missing the woman who made me. When I get old and infirm, I hope my kids will remember to play this music for me. I don't know that they will, they speak no Asian languages and cannot, perhaps, understand how the most integrated migrants feel deep attachments to their past lives. And how their old music makes them young again before the light goes out and death comes to take them away.

Musician, actress, songwriter, producer

The First Time Ever I Saw Your Face by Roberta Flack

For me music isn't just about songs, though as a songwriter I sure appreciate a good song, it's about where, when and what context you first heard a particular piece of music in and although there are a thousands songs I could name that have affected my life positively, if I had to name one piece of music that profoundly changed me, it would be 'Mars' in Holst's 'Planets Suite' because this was the very first piece of music I was encouraged to dance to by my first music teacher Miss Nelson.

This was the beginning for me and I have never looked back.

But if I had to choose a song, it would be 'The First Time Ever I Saw Your Face' sung by Roberta Flack, but it was the way it was placed in the brilliant film *Play Misty For Me* that gave it incredible power. In fact it didn't become a hit until the film was released which proves how a great film, a great story and a great song can make magic happen.

Actor, singer, radio presenter and former lead singer with Manfred Mann.

I've Never Been in Love Before

On 18th January 1982 I was in the first-night audience for *Guys And Dolls* at the National Theatre, thanks to the generosity of its director, Richard Eyre. It was so wonderful, I couldn't even tell him how wonderful. Then a few weeks later, he told me his next production would be *The Beggar's Opera* and asked if I'd be interested in playing Macheath. By the spring of that year, I'd joined the company, and then in the autumn I took over the part of Sky Masterson in *Guys And Dolls* as well. For most of 1983, I found myself evening after evening gazing into the beautiful eyes of Sarah Brown (Fiona Hendley) and singing the wonderful music of Frank Loesser, my favourite moment being the segue from 'My Time Of Day' into 'I've Never Been In Love Before', which becomes a duet as Sarah joins Sky in confessing the 'helpless haze' of love.

Fast forward to 16th December 1984, at All Souls Church, Langham Place, in London's West End; Fiona and I are celebrating our marriage with family, friends and a large proportion of the cast of those two great shows – including Sir Richard Eyre. The Director of Music at All Souls (and of The

All Souls Orchestra) Noel Tredinnick is in charge of the music for the service, and as Fiona and I walk back down the aisle together, what rings out from the organ? No Wedding March from Lohengrin for us; it's 'I've Never Been In Love Before'. 26 years on, it's a beautiful and powerful memory-song for us.

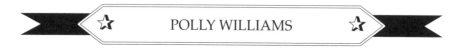

POLLY WILLIAMS

Novelist and journalist

Heroes by David Bowie

My favourite song is; 'Heroes' by David Bowie.

It reminds me of being a teenager, growing up in Oxford, and dreaming of the love of my life who I hadn't met yet! Many floppy-haired, unsuitable men later … no, I didn't find anyone worthy of it for many more years. It still brings a lump to my throat though. Fantastic.

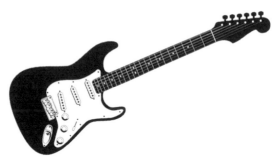

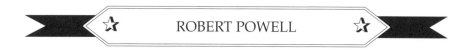

ROBERT POWELL

Actor

Don't Think Twice, It's Alright by Bob Dylan.

Dylan was the single biggest influence on my musical life when I was a young man. I have all his albums and each track brings back memories of where and when.

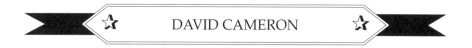

DAVID CAMERON

Prime Minister of the UK

Tangled up in Blue by Bob Dylan

The live version of Bob Dylan's 'Tangled Up In Blue' would be the song I would take to a desert island. The sound of the audience and Dylan's rasping voice would make me feel less lonely.

Novelist

You'll Never Walk Alone by Gerry and The Pacemakers.

A famously iconic song for Liverpool football supporters all over the world, but one which holds huge importance for me too. Kind of ironic considering I support a rival team. But it's a song that never fails to raise a smile for me because it reminds me of the very first time I met the love of my life.

Manchester City F.C. – the Blues. My team, and the real Manchester team, not the corporate one with the stroppy millionaires and pretty boys with changing hairstyles. With Manchester City – it's about the football. Unfortunately, it's also about results, and it is here that the blue half of Manchester have typically fallen short. City are consistent only in their inconsistency, but this is part of the reason their fans love them. They are passionate, unpredictable and always entertaining.

However, on one particular evening back in the spring of 1995 as I sat watching a game with friends in a Dublin pub, another team were doing the entertaining. It wasn't even half-time, and already Liverpool were hammering City 3-0. Fully decked out in sky-blue City regalia – a figure of fun to other football supporters, but well used to the jeering, I didn't give up hope. With City, you never give up hope.

I looked up as a small group sat down at the recently-vacated table alongside ours. 'I think you're backing the also-ran,' one guy called out. I looked up, fully prepared to put the jeering so-and-so in his place but stopped short, unprepared for the sight of his alarmingly bright blue eyes and his warm, easygoing expression.

'We'll get them back in the second half – it's not over yet,' I answered defiantly, but rather shakily, my earlier composure fading at his lazy grin and the teasing challenge in his eyes. He gave a little smile, shrugged and said no more. The second half of the game began. My boys battled with everything they had but soon it was 4-0. I shook my head and stole a sideways glance at my tormentor, seeing him stifle a grin as he stared at the television, pretending not to notice me.

Then, things began to seriously disintegrate as City had a perfectly good goal disallowed. I put my head in my hands.

"It could be worse," he teased, passing by me on his way to the bar and soon enough, it was. City had a player sent off and a penalty awarded. If this went in, I was going home.

The Liverpool player stepped up to take the kick. I turned my head away and closed my eyes; unable to watch what I knew would be the inevitable, as Robbie Fowler rarely missed penalties. The referee blew his whistle and, for me, time stood still. Then there was a loud roar, and I knew it was all over. I groaned inwardly. 5-0! How could I ever live this down? 'He's missed it,' said a disbelieving voice from beside me – his voice.

"What?" I whispered, equally disbelieving, eyes wide as I looked from the TV screen, to him and back. And the player had missed it, or more importantly, our goalkeeper had saved it!

"Yes!" I cried out, and in the excitement of moment, grabbed the good-looking stranger and gave him a delighted hug. Then, instantly realising what I had done, I pulled away, slightly embarrassed.

"Well, City fans don't normally have much to celebrate – you might as well enjoy it while you can!" he laughed, not in the least bit put out.

His name was Kevin, and the reason he was having so much fun teasing me that night was because he was a life-long Liverpool fan, and had been totally taken aback by my City allegiance. I told him that not all women were interested in football merely because of sallow-skinned, fiery Italians or long-haired Frenchmen with taut, muscular thighs. For most of us, it was about the football. He remained sceptical until we began what turned into an evening-long argument about the wizardry of Brazilian football, the advantages and disadvantages of Roy Keane's temperament (years later, I was to be proved right) and whether or not Manchester United (yawn) would sweep the board in the competitions again that season.

And at the end of the game, when he and the other Liverpool supporters celebrated their win with a rousing rendition of 'You'll Never Walk Alone', he urged me to join in.

Soon after, we began seeing one another on a regular basis. I was in heaven. Finally, someone who shared my passion for 'The Beautiful Game', someone who understood the ferocious rivalry between the red and blue sides of a famous footballing city, someone who would quite happily spend Saturday afternoons waiting for the day's football results to come in on the sports channels, someone who understood the offside rule, and cursed diabolical refereeing decisions.

1998 was a big year for football. It was the year the World Cup finals took place in France, the year David Beckham was vilified for being sent off in the game against Argentina, the year Zinedine Zidane enthralled the world with his awe-inspiring talent, ensuring France lifted the most coveted trophy in football.

It was also the year Kevin proposed. We've been married ten years now and have just had a baby daughter. Seems that when it came to us, the famous Liverpool anthem we sang together that night back in 1995 turned out to be prophetic in many ways.

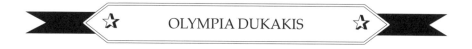

OLYMPIA DUKAKIS

Actress

My mother would always sing Greek songs together and then she couldn't remember them. I thought that I should stop singing them but my son told me that she was affected by the music. And so I sang to her until she died and I'm glad I did. Music was important to both of us.

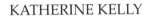

KATHERINE KELLY

Actress, who plays Becky McDonald in Coronation Street

The Fields of Athenry

I have so many favourite songs. I grew up in a house filled with music and my favourite songs are my favourite songs because I associate them with an event or feeling!!!

I have chosen the 'Fields of Athenry'. It is a beautiful old Irish ballad set during the Great Irish Famine. The lyrics are very depressing actually! But the memories I associate with it aren't. When I hear this song it transports me back to my childhood summers spent in Ireland. My dad is Irish and I think of him and my brothers singing and playing their guitars with our cousins in Kerry. This song fills me with a sense of history and hope. I always feel really emotional when I hear it, especially if my family are singing it, but it's a good emotion!

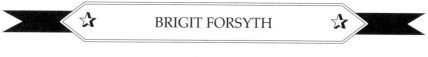

BRIGIT FORSYTH

Actress

You Should be Dancing by The Bee-Gees

My song is 'You Should be Dancing' by The Bee-Gees, as it always makes me get up and dance.

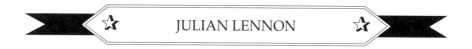

JULIAN LENNON

Musician/songwriter/photographer

Whiter Shade of Pale by Procol Harum

The song 'Whiter Shade of Pale' by Procol Harum resonates with an interesting memory for me as it was my very first introduction to 'rock and roll'!

I was 5 years old when I was taken by my father to the Rolling Stones' 'Rock and Roll Circus' recording. This song was playing as we entered through a long hallway towards a purple light; we then had to go through a curtain, and beyond that were all these crazy-looking people, including one terrifying clown that left me with a lifelong fear of them!

Burlesque artist, model and actress

Love is a Losing Game by Amy Winehouse

One of my favourite recent musical memories is of a song called 'Love is a Losing Game' by Amy Winehouse. As a fan of the blues artists of the early and mid 20th century, when I first heard Amy Winehouse, I immediately became enthralled with her music. One night I was out in London with my sisters, my best friend and my mother, and I met Amy. She was behind the bar, fixing her own drink, and she said to me 'would you like to come over to my house and I can play some songs for you?' Of course we followed her to her house, which was a right mess, but she sat there cross-legged in the middle of the floor in her dishevelled living room, drinking from a giant jug of sake she said she had received as a gift, and she played guitar and sang so soulfully and so perfectly, song after song, just for us. She sang her own songs, but also some very obscure 1930s songs, and even some of my mother's favourite 60s songs, songs I had never even heard of! I will never forget her knowledge of music, and the beauty, tragedy and truth that came from her own inimitable voice, a voice with something so much more than a technically talented pop songstress. I was so moved by her, and what I will always believe is that she is the closest thing our generation will ever have to a legend like Billie Holiday.

Radio and TV presenter

The Long and Winding Road by The Beatles

I grew up on a farm in Sussex which was in a very picturesque setting with the river Arun running through it. It was run by my grandfather and was in a very remote spot, approached by a long and winding road.

When I was fifteen my grandfather retired, the farm was sold and I thought I would never go back there again. Five years ago I discovered that a friend of mine, who had been a member of the band Marmalade, was living in a very old house on the farm. My wife and I went to visit him and I at last returned to the farm I hadn`t seen for over fifty years . Little more than a year later he moved on and I bought the house.

Every time I head back to the farm the song the Beatles wrote, 'The Long And Winding Road', goes through my mind. My life has taken me on a long and winding road and now, finally, I am back home.

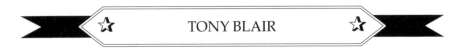

TONY BLAIR

Former Prime Minister of the UK

Jerusalem

Although I enjoy a variety of music, my favourite hymn is 'Jerusalem'.

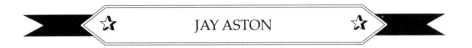

JAY ASTON

Singer and former member of Bucks Fizz

Cinderella Rockefella by Esther and Abi Ofarim

The first record I bought was called 'Cinderella Rockefella'.

It was by Esther and Abi Ofarim and I used to dance around my front room till I was dizzy.

It started with 'You're a lady, you're a lady .... that I love'

My mum used to come out from the kitchen and watch me twirl, I was about seven.

Novelist

Times Like These by Foo Fighters

No matter how grey the day in London, 'Times Like These' by Foo Fighters brings back the sunshine with its opening bar. It takes me straight to the spring of 2004, when I spent a couple of months living in Santa Monica in Los Angeles while finishing a book. I had three CDs in my hire car and 'One By One' was undoubtedly my favourite soundtrack for a drive up the coast. One particular morning, while singing along somewhat more exuberantly than usual, I turned my car into the path of an oncoming fire engine. For a moment I'd forgotten to drive on the 'wrong' side of the road. The fire engine braked, thank goodness, leaving me perfectly unharmed if a little shaken. You'd think that would have taken the edge off 'Times Like These' but a day later I was singing it again, feeling all the more strongly – perhaps thanks to my near-death experience – that I had to be in the moment, there are no dress rehearsals, ya-da, ya-da, ya-da … As the song says: It's times like these you learn to live again. Towards the end of my Santa Monica sojourn, my best friend Guy visited and together we drove up Highway 1 to San Francisco. 'Times Like These' especially brings to mind snapshots from Guy's week in California: his knock-kneed stance as we learned to roller-blade, the smile on a face of a sea otter at the aquarium in Monterey, the scary motel at Ragged Point where I convinced myself that the proprietor was a serial killer. It brings to mind an afternoon at the Getty Museum, finding the building more interesting than the art. It's the boat ride to Alcatraz. It's drinks on the Sunset Strip. It's the unexpected upgrade on the flight back to London. It's one of the happiest times of my life and hearing it makes me remember, even on the darkest day, that there's more sunshine to come.

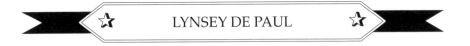

LYNSEY DE PAUL

Singer, songwriter and actress

The Folks Who Live on the Hill

I have always loved the song 'The Folks Who Live On The Hill', which was written long before I was born by Oscar Hammerstein and Jerome Kern. It has a wonderful, meandering melody, a beautiful chord structure and one of the most nostalgic lyrics ever written about two people. There is a pianist in a certain restaurant I sometimes go to and, as soon as I appear, he plays the song because he knows how much I love it. It never fails to move me to tears and make me smile at the same time.

Barrister and wife of former Prime Minister Tony Blair

Que Sera Sera

When I was just two years old, I was moved from Liverpool where I had been living with my paternal grandparents, to live with my mum and dad in Stoke Newington, London where my parents were working as actors and where my sister Lyndsey had just been born. I was not at all happy to be moved from a place where I was the centre of attention and I missed my grandma. Less than a year later I was back with my grandparents in Liverpool and this time with my mother and sister, but without my father. While I was away from Liverpool, I sent a message on a reel to reel tape recorder to my grandma of me singing 'Que Sera Sera'. Whenever I hear the song it reminds me of her and of my family and how you can never predict where life will take you.

Novelist

Jump by Van Halen

I mused upon all the songs that make my heart twang, stomach loop or eyes stream with tears and then I thought, if I was going to give someone a memory, I'd like it to be a happy, possibly faintly ridiculous, one. And so I give you 'Jump' by Van Halen:

It was 1994 and my best friend Emily and I were in Paris to see the Chippendales. I realise that sounds wrong on so many counts – why would anyone visit this most chic and romantic of cities to watch American body-builders flex their oil-varnished physiques? Why take a plane to see them at all? Well, I'd actually interviewed the guys for a magazine and become pally with one of the performers – a raven-maned dancer named Murray. He would often get us free tickets to the London show – *A Musical with Muscle* – which proved to be quite a revelation for two girls with unfashionably retro musical tastes. We had always been solely devoted to the most genteel of crooners – Doris Day, Andy Williams, Julio Iglesias… Suddenly we were 'exposed' to the world of straggly-haired rockers and found ourselves joyfully fist-pumping the air to Queen and Def Leppard. After about the third show we lost interest in ogling the men on stage and instead would go along as a kind of lavish karaoke experience so we could belt out 'We Will Rock You' and 'Pour Some Sugar on Me'. Not quite sing-a-long *The Sound of Music* but these thrusting anthems proved addictive and so when the show shifted to Paris, so did we. For a weekend, at least.

Murray had arranged to meet us at the ultra-swish nightclub Les Bains Douches and I remember as we were leaving our poky Montmartre hotel the grumpy man on reception asked where we were headed and scoffed when we told him – 'You'll never get in,' he grunted. 'All the models go there.' Of course we just took this as a challenge on behalf of all the ordinary-looking girls of the world. (Little did he know that Emily has the kind of flirtation skills that could out-do Adriana Lima in a negligee.)

But when the bouncer waved us in (Arc de Triumph!) it turned out that the reception guy was at least half right – it was full of models and thus far too posy for our taste (nothing irritates Emily more than blank-faced beauties gazing around the room waiting for someone to come up and admire them/ buy them something). We said we'd catch up with Murray the next night and left in search of something more casual and that's when we heard the thump-thump-boom coming from a basement cavern playing 80s music. We burrowed into the darkness and began dancing, released from the need to look cool, we even incorporated a few moves we'd learned from the Chippendales. And then that instantly recognisable synth opening struck up. As we'd done a dozen times that evening we gasped, 'Oh my god, I love this song!' and then decided to clamber up on to the nearby ledge so we could take the upcoming chorus literally. As Eddie Van Halen roared, 'Might as well JUMP!' so we sprang upward, Emily obviously with more gusto than me – she struck her head on the low ceiling beam and fell, leaden and unconscious, to the floor.

It took a while to revive her but even as an egg-shaped swelling began to protrude from her forehead she began to giggle. Soon the pair of us were helpless with laughter. I don't think the hysteria abated until we flew home.

Every time I hear that song now I think of that moment and grin to myself, which perhaps I wouldn't do had it been my skull getting the clunking. What I really love about it is that it instantly transports me back to a time when I lived with such fanciful abandon. The older I get the more wary I become – I weigh up the pros, cons and consequences before I do anything. It's such a bore. But every now and again when I'm teetering on the brink of trying something new or about to back away from a situation due to feeble, middle-aged nerves I hear Van Halen dare me, 'MIGHT AS WELL JUMP!'

And then I do.

(After a quick cautionary assessment of the ceiling.)

TV presenter and journalist

Feelin' Hot Hot Hot

The year was 1984 and I was about to leave the country that had been home for most of my life thus far. At fourteen, and having moved many times, I was enjoying being back 'home' in Trinidad, and wasn't looking forward to the idea of starting again at another new school, and making more new friends in the UK, the country of my birth. Carnival had always played a huge part in our life, from kiddie parties through to teenage 'limes' it was, and still is, the biggest time of year in Trinidad. So, for the last time, we took to the streets of Port-of-Spain as a family, to chip behind the floats and the bands. The costumes were amazing, and the sweet sound of steel band filled the air, fighting above the racket of DJ's blaring out the latest soca tunes. The song that dominated that year was 'Feelin' Hot Hot Hot'. I danced down the dusty streets of Port-of-Spain, my sister and I laughing at the pink and sweating tourists jiggling alongside us. And every time I hear that song I am transported back to a time when I was young, the sun was hot, and I was a Trini girl, instead of the pink, sweating tourist that I have become.

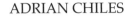

TV presenter, writer and West Bromwich Albion supporter

Don't You Want Me by The Human League

It's not even a song I particularly like but it instantly transports me back to a time and place more than any other. It was the early eighties and it seemed to be played every other track on the radio. It was winter and it snowed and, praise be, they shut the school for the day. Joy. My mate Rich had a small snooker table in the basement of his house. So we just played snooker all day. Two pubescent boys playing snooker intensely and, just as intensely, discussing girls who'd never reciprocate our interest. We knew it, but we were off school for the day, so we were happy.

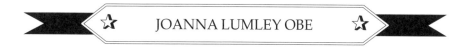

Actress and author

Stardust by Nat King Cole

My favourite song is Nat King Cole singing 'Stardust' as it reminds me of being a child in the Far East.

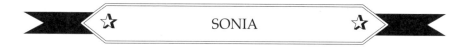

SONIA

Singer, songwriter and actress

Let's Wait a While by Janet Jackson

The song that gives me my fondest memory is 'Let's Wait a While' by Janet Jackson. Me and my husband had our first dance together to this song when we were both sixteen, we had just met each other that night at the after-show party for the school play I was in. Twenty-three years later we are still together and have a three-month baby girl. I have to thank that song for us meeting it's also such a lovely song.

Journalist and TV presenter

Lamb by Gorecki Band

Quite an obscure song but the most evocative and emotional song I've ever heard. When I hear it now, it reminds me of university and meeting my wife. The words are compelling and the voice is ethereal in sound. It also led me to discovering the composer Gorecki, who has written some extraordinary pieces of work – listen to it, it will change your life! It changed mine.

DAME MARY PETERS DBE

Former athlete and gold Olympic medalist

Chariots of Fire

'Chariots of Fire' stirs memories for me of competing in three Olympic Games in the days when we were all amateurs striving for success for our country.

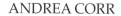
Singer, songwriter and actress

State of Independence by Donna Summer

My brother Jim used to go away for months touring with (would you believe it?!) a family band consisting of three girls and a boy. When he would come home he would bring records that the girls in that band practised with vocally. I, being ten years younger, was naturally keen on impressing him with my voice when he would return and would sing and practise all the days long. A labour of love for me. The song I remember and love to this day is 'State of Independence' by Donna Summer … one of the best records ever recorded I believe, and the memory it evokes is that of myself singing along with it in the living room while my mother, peeling the potatoes at the kitchen sink crying, missing my brother, as that year he could not make it home for Christmas.

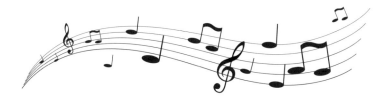

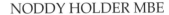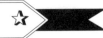

NODDY HOLDER MBE

Musician, actor and former lead singer with Slade

You Made Me Love You by Al Jolson

The song is 'You Made Me Love You' by Al Jolson. This is the song that my dad always sang to my mum when he was feeling in a romantic mood, either at home or in the working men's clubs. It also helps me remember big family get-togethers from when I was a kid, and show-offs would get up and do a song after a few wee drinkies!

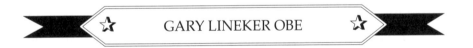

GARY LINEKER OBE

TV sports presenter and former professional footballer

Nessun Dorma by Luciano Pavarotti

A very evocative song for me is Pavarotti's rendition of 'Nessun Dorma' – it is a truly wonderful piece of music in itself, but also brings back so many memories of the 1990 World Cup.

CARMEN REID

Author

I'm on My Way by The Proclaimers.

I just love the downright infectious happiness of this song. This is a hand-clapping, foot-tapping, boogie-along song. It was the theme tune to *Shrek*, so I've belted it out at top volume in the car with my children. Happy days! When I was moving back to Scotland from London, it came on the radio and seemed like a good omen. I remember dancing to it at my sister's wedding – everyone singing along. A song like this is the essence of a Scottish party and you've not really partied till you've partied in Scotland, preferably with exuberant men in swinging kilts! The words present a lovely idea: that we're all on our way from misery to happiness. If I'm feeling miserable, I'll play this and realise that there's a simple way to travel back to happiness again.

Actress

You Were Meant For Me

I've always loved the song anyway but this little incident, which took place a while back, made it into a memory.

I was walking along, near where I live, when I saw a young fellow walking towards me. When he was near, he didn't veer away but came right up to me. I thought he was going to ask for my autograph. Instead, he looked into my eyes and began to sing. I kept very still, like you might if a lion approached you. He was singing 'You Were Meant For Me'. He sang the whole song, quietly and sweetly, slowing up on the last phrase to make a good finish. If we had been Fred and Ginger, we would have begun to sway and then gone into our dance. Instead, I smiled. He smiled back and sort of bowed awkwardly, then turned and walked away. I knew how he felt. He obviously adored the song so much that he'd had to sing it to someone or he'd burst.

The whole thing was so nonsensical and sweet, and I think of it whenever I hear the song.

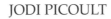

Novelist

Tears in Heaven by Eric Clapton

One song that always stops me in my tracks is 'Tears In Heaven' by Eric Clapton. When it came out, I was a new mother – quite young – and quite unprepared for a very colicky son. I am not sure what it was about that song, but whenever it played on the radio Kyle would stop wailing and just listen. I knew that the song had been written by Clapton for his own son, who'd died in an accident – and there was something about my baby boy going still at the sound of the melody and the lyrics written for another little boy that never failed to make my heart catch.

Actor, musician,

Car Wash by Rose Royce

My song has to be 'Car Wash' by Rose Royce.

I was fifteen and it was the first time I had been allowed out to a nightclub by my parents. My mates and I were all nearly six foot by now and starting to see the first signs of stubble and I had recently been pissed for the very first time on Pernod and lemonade. The big nightclub in the mid seventies was The Lyceum in London's Covent Garden, a big old ballroom where up to 1500 people would gather on a Wednesday night to dance to Donna Summer, KC and the Sunshine Band and George McCrea. As I walked into the guilded entrance on that first night and bought my ticket, I felt my stomach roll with nerves, the place had everything a fifteen-year-old boy could want …. Alcohol, girls and music, but it wasn't till I opened the swing doors that led into the main room of the club that I realised how good that music was. Just as I started my way down the gold steps, the hand clap sequence to Rose Royce's track 'Car Wash' started fading in through the giant PA system at the front of the stage, and it got louder, louder and louder, I had never heard music played like this before, the bass rattling my bones and the treble taking out my inner ear. It was wonderful. I will never forget that feeling, or that record.

Actress

Summertime

'Summertime' from Gershwin's *Porgy and Bess* is a song that brings back a lot of happy memories for me. My mother was an actress before my sisters and I were born (there are four of us altogether) and she was always singing. This was a particular favourite of my father's and she used to sing it so beautifully. Wherever the rest of us were in the house, we'd hear her and all join in whether we were in the bath or doing homework or whatever, until the whole family was singing. It's a song that just reminds me of my younger days and a very happy childhood.

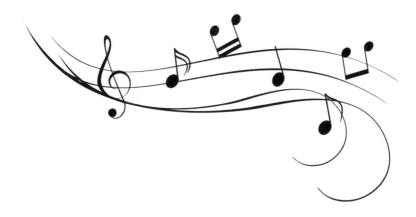

HANNAH WATERMAN

Actress

Band on the Run by Wings

One of my earliest memories is being in an open-topped sports car with my mum and 'Band on the Run' playing at full volume while me, my mum, and sister all sang along. It was exhilarating and felt such fun.

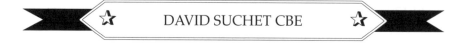

DAVID SUCHET CBE

Actor

When I Fall in Love by Nat King Cole

I sang this song to a young girl that I had fallen in love with. We were both acting at The Belgrade Theatre, Coventry. It was our first date. The year was 1972. Four years later we married. Sheila is still my wife!

Lawyer, business woman and patron of various charities

My Way by Frank Sinatra

I love the idea of donating a song and a memory. There is nothing like a song to evoke atmosphere: almost like a time capsule to the past. My song is – of course – 'My Way' as sung by Frank Sinatra, although it has been sung by all the greats over time. I just love 'Old Blue Eyes' and the rich resonance of his voice always gives me a sense of the power of the human spirit to overcome adversity whenever I hear this song. London is also my favourite city and when I discovered the Sid Vicious version of the song from the 'Punk Rock' era – it just summed up all my impressions of England. The same indomitable spirit which the English bring to football – I try to bring to living my life – that is like the song says, 'Doing it My Way'.

151

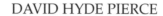

DAVID HYDE PIERCE

Actor

Dancing Cheek to Cheek

'Dancing Cheek to Cheek' holds great memories for me. My mum and dad were wonderful ballroom dancers, and after nearly fifty years together, they danced as one person – not as flashy as Fred and Ginger, but, in a quiet way, just as good.

The song reminds me of them at their happiest, and the opening lyric; 'Heaven, I'm in heaven' always makes me think that's where they're dancing now.

CHRIS TARRANT OBE

TV and radio presenter

Yesterday by The Beatles

My favourite song is The Beatles' 'Yesterday' as it evokes memories of my childhood and of growing up.

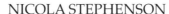
Actress

Midnight Train to Georgia by Gladys Knight and the Pips

The song that springs to mind, there are so many, is 'Midnight Train To Georgia' by Gladys Knight and the Pips. It was on a 'best of' album which my mum owned and it brings back a memory of me sitting on the bed, aged 5, watching my pretty, glamorous mummy get ready with her false eyelashes and blue denim platform boots. Later in life, in the drunken nights out of my twenties, it became a karaoke favourite and so reminds me of many a happy time with my two best friends Angela Griffin and Lisa Faulkner. Now in my thirties it is still being played as I dance around my kitchen with my two daughters Iris and Esme. I hope they grow up with it reminding them of me.

Head of School of Psychological Sciences, University of Manchester, author and former Big Brother psychologist

Mandolin Wind by Rod Stewart

For good psychological reasons, no doubt, I find 'Mandolin Wind' by Rod Stewart to be very evocative of a particular place and a particular time. It was the summer before I went to university and I had hitch-hiked to London to sleep rough in one or other of the London parks, as many young Irishmen were then prone to do; it was a city that I hardly knew. The song was playing on the radio of the car in which I was travelling. The driver let me out on Church Street, Kensington because that is where he was travelling to himself, and a stunning-looking man walked past with his jeans tucked into his boots. He was the first person I saw that day. It was such a glamorous and compelling image and I thought to myself 'So this is London'. I thought that all of London must be like High Street Ken, with Biba and its ultra trendy boutiques. I could almost feel my past leaving my body, like some departing astral spirit, and I could feel myself being reborn at that very moment in time. This would be the new trendy me, the old me, fashioned in the grey streets of Belfast, gone for ever. (Of course, life was not as simple as that, but that's how it all felt, on that great optimistic, life-changing day). It is such an odd and distinctive memory from thirty odd years ago that has not been degraded or diminished by time. The fashion was for tight, suede jackets and boots in interesting and unusual colours and I fell in love with a suede jacket and green boots, neither of which I could afford, so I had to hitch-hike back to London the following week to get the coat. The boots had to be saved for and bought much later. I can sit back now and smell that coat as if it is in front of me. I just have to hum that tune, even in my head, and I am back to that afternoon with the sun shining, and my dreams of new exotic personal images, of change, of possible worlds, just out there, hopefully soon to be within reach. That is how powerful some songs can be.

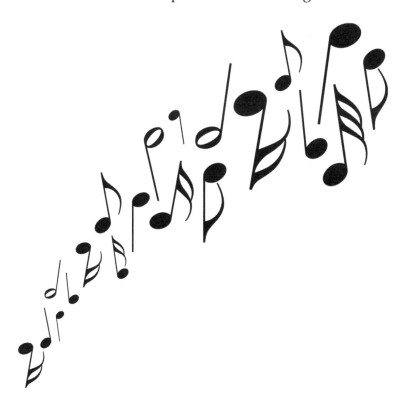

Food writer

Groove is in the Heart by Dee Lite

I would like to pretend that my favourite musical memory was some obscure, cerebral classical piece. Or haunting aria, warbled by a long dead maestro. This would make me seem more learned and cultured than I really am. But this isn't Desert Island Discs, so I can be entirely honest. 'Groove is in The Heart' is a perfect piece of bubblegum dance pop, written and performed by Dee Lite at the very dawn of the nineties. I could bang on about the Herbie Hancock samples or the fact that Funkadelic legend Bootsy Collins strummed bass guitar, as well as providing some of the backing vocals. But really, this is a song that never fails to make me happy. It reminds me of my teenage years, of cheap booze, boundless optimism and the endless summer nights of school holidays. And, of course, the pretty girls who seemed distinctly unimpressed by my clumsy, feverish dancing. Great video, fine song and it still sends a shiver of visceral joy straight up my spine.

Broadcaster/journalist/author

Thanks for the Memory by Bob Hope

The song 'Thanks For The Memory' has a particular resonance for me. I loved it when I first heard it sung by Bob Hope in a black and white movie, when I was a snotty kid on the back row of a cinema in Yorkshire. Then in 1981 at the end of my first stint with the BBC with the talk show, Bob Hope sung a specially amended version to wave me farewell. When I finally retired from the talk show in 2007, Dame Judi Dench sang the song during my farewell programme.

Bob Hope is one thing, but to be serenaded by Dame Judi quite another. So it's a song with a very special significance in my life.

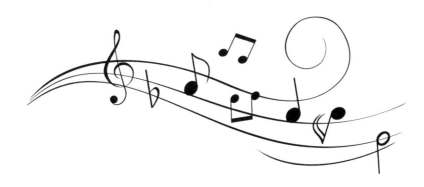

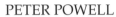

PETER POWELL

Former DJ and chairman of the James Grant Media Group

Love and Emotion by Joan Armatrading

'Love and Emotion' by Joan Armatrading was the last record I played on Radio 1 when I left in 1988 and indeed the last record I have ever played in public. Raw, beautiful and real it still sends a shiver down my back. It's one of those rare songs which puts your life on hold for a few minutes followed by a few seconds peace and quiet when it finishes. Everyone in the world needs moments like that.

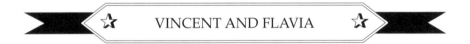

VINCENT AND FLAVIA

Professional dancers and stars of Strictly Come Dancing

Quejas de Bandoneon by Astor Piazolla

It was the first Argentine Tango song which we choreographed for our first show dance, so it has a huge amount of meaning to us, we will never get bored of dancing it.

Musician, singer

Aladdin Sane by David Bowie

Because I'm a musician, music tends not to evoke memories for me as I play so much music all the time.

Strange then, that the other day I was playing Bowie's 'Aladdin Sane' album, and all these memories came back of when I was too young to analyse the record, but just enjoyed the feeling I had of Bowie's invention of 'The Spiders From Mars', a fictitious band from another planet, that started on the Ziggy Stardust album.

On this track, 'Drive In Saturday', it's the future and they are watching old movies from Earth, and trying to piece together what human life was like on Earth circa the 50s–60s... and everyone's name seemed to be 'Buddy'!

Because I was more into soul music even then, Bowie's music seemed new and fresh, and more easily put images in my head, as opposed to soul music that just stirred my emotions.

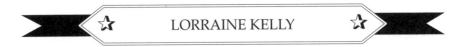

LORRAINE KELLY

TV presenter and journalist

Constant Craving by k.d. lang

My favourite song is 'Constant Craving' by k.d. lang – it makes me think of holidays in the sunshine.

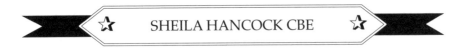

SHEILA HANCOCK CBE

Actress and author

The Sun Has Got His Hat On

'The Sun Has Got His Hat On' reminds me of my husband (the late John Thaw) who used it to cheer us and himself up.

Radio host, TV presenter and writer

The Way You Look Tonight by Fred Astaire

My song would be 'The Way You Look Tonight'. Written by Jerome Kern and Dorothy Fields, Fred Astaire sang the song in Swing Time. Astaire reminds me so much of my grandfather, both in looks and the fact that in most photographs I have of my grandfather he's wearing black tie and tails. One photograph even has him dancing on a packed dancefloor (in black tie) with a wooden chair!

An evocative song (that conjures up an era that I never saw) from the composer of 'Smoke Gets in Your Eyes' and 'Ol' Man River'.

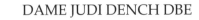

DAME JUDI DENCH DBE

Actress, author, director

You Have Cast Your Shadow on the Sea

One of my favourite songs is called 'You Have Cast Your Shadow on the Sea' and it comes from the musical *The Boys from Syracuse*. I directed this show at the Open Air Theatre in Regent's Park in 1991. I have always liked the song, even before I directed the musical, but now it reminds me of a very happy time spent at the theatre.

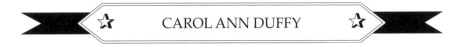

CAROL ANN DUFFY

The Poet Laureate

Danny Boy by Frederick Weatherly

Every time I hear this song it reminds me of my mum. It brings back happy memories. When she passed away we had a soprano sing it at her funeral.

Novelist

We Are the Champions by Queen

The song that means most to me is 'We Are the Champions', sung by Freddie Mercury of Queen, my all-time favourite band.

This song is extra-special because in 1990 I was working for a boss who had an Olympic gold medal in emotional bullying, and by the end of another day of being on the receiving end of this I was exhausted.

On the way home, I'd always put Queen on the stereo of my ancient Vauxhall Cavalier and, as I drove home through the dusk, I'd be cheered and re-energised by the band that represents the ultimate in British glam rock. By the time the tape got to 'We Are the Champions', I'd have forgotten all about the trials and tribulations of the day. As I walked into the house to start again, to turn on the washing machine and get the dinner going, I'd still be wearing my silver platform heels, and still be strutting my stuff with Freddie and the band. So thank you, Freddie, wherever you are now, for always making me feel better about myself, the universe and everything. Twenty years later, a few minutes of Queen on my CD player makes me believe that, however badly things are going, I'm going to win through. It's a kind of magic!

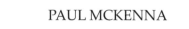
Hypnotist and self improvement author

A Song for You by Donny Hathaway

One of my favourites is 'A Song for You' by Donny Hathaway
(written by Leon Russell). It reminds me of listening to
songs late at night with friends, having conversations about
everything and anything, laughing and sharing funny stories.
Love and friends to me are amongst the most important things
in life. I hope the song touches you too.

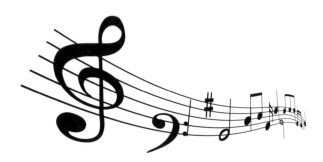

Interior designer and TV presenter

Kodachrome by Simon and Garfunkel

My song is 'Kodachrome' by Simon and Garfunkel.

It's a song that is immediately uplifting and I have it as an instant, feel good, track in the car and no matter how tough the day is I just can't help sing along, in fact I belt it out usually, it's a ray of sunshine. The lyrics refer to colours being brighter and as an interior designer that's exactly what I'm trying to do with people's lives, simply to make a black and white world seem brighter. It's not a serious tune and it's certainly a bit of a closet confession, but I love the harmonies of Simon and Garfunkel and many of their tracks take me back to my happy childhood where my sisters would tap out the songs on the piano at home.

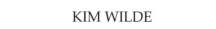

KIM WILDE

Singer, author and TV presenter

My Eyes Adored You by Frankie Valli and the Four Seasons.

This song transports me back to my school days in the 70s when my oldest friend Clare and I would wait for the school coach to arrive at the bottom of our lane. I was madly in love with a boy who used to get on the bus at the next stop in Datchworth, but this worship was just from afar, just like the words in the song. I must have been around thirteen or fourteen years old, and then many years later we met bizarrely on the Chris Evans show, *Don't Forget your Toothbrush*. Chris had flown him all the way from Ireland to see me! Life can be very strange and wonderful sometimes.

TV presenter

Moonlight Serenade by The Glenn Miller Orchestra

I love any Glenn Miller song, particularly 'Moonlight Serenade' as it reminds me of my grandad, he also suffers from Alzheimer's. He is a war hero and a very special man. At 93 he still delights me with his stories of his time during the war, meeting my wonderful grandmother and memories of his comrades.

☆ EDWARD FOX OBE ☆

Actor

Some Enchanted Evening by Ezio Pinza

My good musical memory, being so many, is of 'Some Enchanted Evening' from the musical *South Pacific* and sung by the original artist Ezio Pinza. This is everything that romantic singing should be.

Novelist

Our Love is Here to Stay by Gene Kelly

Almost my favourite tune in the world is Gene Kelly singing, 'Our Love is Here to Stay' it goes, 'The Rockies may crumble, Gibraltar may tumble, they're only made of clay, but our love is here to stay'.

I remember I went to France one year with my parents and Gene Kelly had just come out in the film *An American in Paris* in which he sang the song. The lift wasn't working in the hotel so we walked up all these flights of stairs and from all levels I used to hear my father or mother singing different bits about The Rockies crumbling and Gibraltar may tumble but our love is here to stay'. It's such a beautiful tune. I love Gene Kelly's voice: that wonderful purring softness. I was madly in love with him when I was a teenager and met him once later in life when he came to a launch party, and he was sweet. I told him what a wonderful song it was.

I also had the song sung as one of my eight records when I went on Desert Island Discs at the end of the seventies with Roy Plomley. And Roy Plomley and I both lived in Putney at the time so we had a wonderful programme, playing this marvellous music, including 'Our Love is Here to Stay' and saying how wonderful Putney was and talking up the prices of our respective houses. It was funny.

168

Author and former Member of Parliament

Penny Lane by The Beatles

My song would be The Beatles 'Penny Lane', because that is where I grew up, in Liverpool. Penny Lane is a real place and the song lists places and faces I can remember well – the pretty nurse selling poppies on a tray, the fireman and his clean machine. It was a bus (formerly tram) terminus about 3 miles from the centre of town, a short walk from home. Paul McCartney, George Harrison and John Lennon all lived nearby too; Paul and George went (like me) to the prestigious Liverpool Institute. I loved the way Paul celebrated ordinary things and people, how he valued our suburban way of life. Our school was closed in the dark days of the 1980s by Militant members of Liverpool City Council, yet another example of how to ruin a city. But now the girls' school is a centre for continuing education for women, and the boys' is the Liverpool Fame Academy producing brilliantly talented youngsters for TV and stage. And Liverpool is a happier, more prosperous place. So life does go on!

Model, fashion designer and TV presenter

Kiss of Life by Sade

My song is by Sade, its called 'Kiss of life'

'There must have been an angel by my side, something heavenly led me to you' is the opening line of this song. It really is how I felt when I met the father of my children, Gabriel. Whenever I hear this song it reminds me of the wonderful, deliriously happy times we had. Now he really is our angel, guiding the kids and me from up above. This is for my two angels, Gabriel and my father John Butcher. x

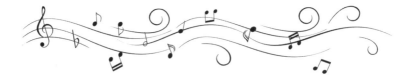

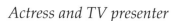
Actress and TV presenter

Strangers in the Night, Something Stupid by Frank and Nancy Sinatra

When my sister Debbie and I were young before our teens, we went on several holidays to the South of England such as Devon, Cornwall and the Isle of Wight. As my dad was the only driver he used to enjoy singing as we went along. Unfortunately his repertoire was rather limited so we used to get repeated renditions of the same songs. The ones I remember best, probably because I heard them the most, were 'Strangers in the Night' and 'Something Stupid'. You can tell he was a big Frank Sinatra fan. In fact not so long ago we were at a karaoke night and he made me get up and sing 'Something Stupid' with him à la Frank and Nancy Sinatra! So when I hear those songs now they bring back the memories of those car journeys but also the happy holidays we had all those years ago.

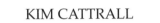
KIM CATTRALL

Actress

I Wanna Hold Your Hand by The Beatles

This reminds me of being allowed to stay up late on a Sunday night to watch The Beatles debut on *The Ed Sullivan Show*. We were supporting the 'boys' from our home town of Liverpool.

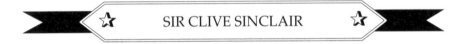
SIR CLIVE SINCLAIR

Inventor, entrepeneur

Shubert songs

I am always deeply moved by Shubert songs as they are so evocative.

Professional dancer and star of Strictly Come Dancing

The Way We Were by Barbra Streisand

Whenever I hear 'The Way We Were' by Barbra Streisand playing it immediately brings back a thousand memories of different countries, cultures and people. I was very lucky that dancing took me all around the world in my twenties and the 'The Way We Were' was the one tune which followed me everywhere, it became the rumba we were requested to perform at amazing events. While performing my favourite dance the rumba, telling a love story, I was communicating to audiences whose language I never spoke and through the song and the moves I connected with people that I, without song and dance, would have never met, let alone connected with. I have had such wonderful feedback from people far far away and hearing that I have left them with a little memory too is, to me, absolutely magnificent! When I play the tune it immediately sends my mind all around the world of so many beautiful memories. 'The Way We Were' will always define my twenties to me!

Musician and actor

Blueberry Hill by Fats Domino

In the 1950s, our house in Jarrow, Tyne and Wear was wired for Rediffusion Radio. We had a choice of the Home Service, Light Programme or Radio Luxembourg.I loved music but couldn't read 'the dots' so I taught myself to play 'by ear'.

One day I heard Fats Domino playing and singing 'Blueberry Hill'. The penny dropped. I thought, I can do that. I nipped into the front room, opened the lid of the upright piano and had a go. It sounded OK.

In closing I am minded of the quote from the banjo player who told me, 'Alan, you start out playing your instrument in you own front room, and that's where you end up.'

I only stopped playing to write this and now I'm going back to practise. Thank you Mr Domino.

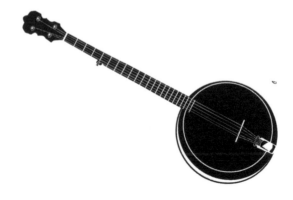

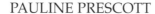

Author and wife of former Deputy Prime Minister John Prescott

How Deep is the Ocean by Marion Montgomery

Music has always played a great part in my life – especially Cole Porter, Gershwin, Glenn Miller and Fats Waller – it is so difficult to choose!

Two songs in particular have been very close to my heart.

My mother and father's favourite song, and also that of my son and daughter-in-law, was 'It Had to be You' – especially the version sung by Frank Sinatra, although Harry Connick Jr's version is fabulous.

The other song is mine, and my husband John's, favourite and with our Golden Wedding Anniversary this year, I think I should choose this because as a love song, for me, the words say it all. The song is 'How Deep is the Ocean' by Marion Montgomery.

Journalist, sportsman and TV presenter

She's Always a Woman to Me by Billy Joel

'She's Always a Woman to Me' by Billy Joel from his 'Scenes from an Italian Restaurant' album.

Whenever I hear that song it reminds me of the time my family drove to the South of France in a Golf convertible. I was ten and my sister was six and my parents had three albums for the cassette machine and this was the favourite. We used to all sing along together. I only have to hear the opening few notes of the song and I can immediately smell the frites, remember all the giggles and the endless searches for hotels in the middle of the night when 'Dad went too far without stopping'.

CAROLINE AHERNE

Actress and writer

A Thing Called Love by Johnny Cash

One of my favourite songs is 'A Thing Called Love' by Johnny Cash. We used this in the 'Queen Of Sheba' Christmas Special episode of *The Royle Family* and it reminds me of the fun we all had during filming. This episode was about the death of Nana and it also reminds me of how special your family are and the memories that they will always leave with you.

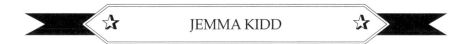 **JEMMA KIDD**

Make-up artist, fashion model and The Countess of Mornington

My Baby Just Cares for Me by Nina Simone

When I moved to New York with my husband (he was my boyfriend at the time) we knew no one and created this new life together. This was the song we played in our new apartment over and over again, it reminds me of the time we had together when it was just the two of us on this great adventure. It was also our wedding song (first dance).

Novelist

Puttin' on the Ritz, Cheek to Cheek,
Let's Face the Music and Dance

Don't make me choose a favourite! But my first movie-loves were Fred Astaire and Ginger Rogers and I remember the absolute joy of discovering them as a teenager. On sunny Sunday afternoons my poor baffled mum would beg me to come outside and sit in the garden with the rest of the family, but nothing could tear me away from the TV, where sparkling black and white romantic comedy combined with heavenly music, and dazzling dance routines held me transfixed.

I had a crush on Fred. I wanted to be Ginger. The sparky dialogue and the chemistry between them was irresistible to me and subsequently had a huge effect on my life – the books I now write borrow heavily from those fabulous feel-good films. I defy anyone to listen to that music and not feel better as a result.

If you have access to the internet, there are endless video clips from the films – I know, because I've just spent an entire afternoon exploring them! Fred and Ginger are there, inside the computer, just waiting for you to press a button. Then they'll spring back to life, as glamorous as ever, and dance – just for you – whenever you like!

Novelist and former politician

Liberty Bell

'Liberty Bell' (better known as the signature tune for *Monty Python's Flying Circus*) always brings back memories of my first election campaign when I was assisting Michael Ancram at Berwick and East Lothian. I drove an ancient Morris through rolling Scottish countryside and dreamed of the day when I would be a candidate myself. That dream came true at the next election when I drove the same Morris around Burnley blaring out the same tune.

ROY HUDD OBE

Comedian, actor, radio host and author

The Hole in the Elephant's Bottom

My favourite song is one I first heard my gran sing. She brought me up and, while other grandchildren may have had pretty lullabys sung to them, my bedtime serenade was a song she'd learned at her mother's knee (or some other low joint!).

The title, if it ever had one, was, and still is 'The Hole In The Elephant's Bottom'.

It made me laugh then and still does today.

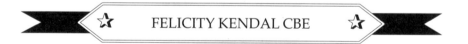

FELICITY KENDAL CBE

Actress

O Mio Babbino Caro by Maria Callas

'O Mio Babbino Caro' from Puccini's opera *Madame Butterfly* – sung by Maria Callas – sublime and moving. It breaks my heart whenever I listen to it.

Actor, writer and TV presenter

Girl of My Best Friend by Elvis Presley

Elvis Presley's 'Girl Of My Best Friend' was playing everywhere in the summer of 1960 when my then girlfriend and I spent two weeks of a summer holiday together. We've been married 44 years now and it still has the power to bring on a burst of soppiness.

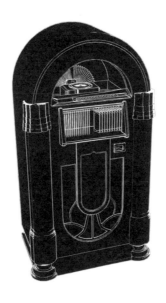

Author

The Very Thought of You

My father and I used to duet to 'The Very Thought of You' at family parties, most of which he spent at the piano. The parties were riotous, and the test of any new boyfriend I brought home was whether he could a) survive and b) join in without looking stupid. The man who was to become my husband not only joined in, but brought his guitar and bothered to learn all the songs, so the song has a double reason to be fondly remembered. Oddly, Lee Marvin's rendition of 'I Was Born Under a Wandering Star' is an instant nostalgia hit as it was at the top of the hit parade in early February 1970, when my husband (now sadly deceased) and I first met. I could go on, as all my family have been or are musicians in one discipline or another, consequently so much music has special memories for me.

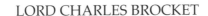

Dance Me to the End of Love by Leonard Cohen

This is such a difficult question as I love music. Music is what puts flavour into the mix that is life, both good and bad. The human brain is an extraordinary creation that has the unique ability to associate even a few bars of a piece of music to an event, exact moment long ago and place that has been buried in the mist of time – and with it all of the emotions that ran through you at that time. I love blues, jazz and rock. When I was younger I thought Leonard Cohen's music was morbid but with age and life experience one realises that he was first a poet and secondly a singer. My choice is 'Dance Me to the End of Love' that tackles so beautifully the frailty of human confidence when touched by real love.

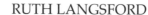

RUTH LANGSFORD

TV presenter

Every Time We Say Goodbye by Ella Fitzgerald

My song is 'Every Time We Say Goodbye' by Ella Fitzgerald because my dad is a big Ella fan and always used to play it to my mum. Now that Dad has Alzheimer's it always makes me cry when I hear it, but it also makes me think of happier times too.

SIR NICK FALDO MBE

Professional golfer and TV presenter

Someone Saved My Life Tonight by Elton John

I've always remembered playing this song on the jukebox down at the pub during the English Amateur Championship at Royal Lytham & St Annes back in 1975. I went on to win the tournament and that was very much the start of my golfing career.

TV presenter

Amazed by Lonestar

I have many songs that evoke memories, but if pushed I would select 'Amazed' by Lonestar.

The words are the perfect description of my beautiful wife, Elizabeth, and when we married last year, July 23rd, I surprised her with my own specially recorded version of the song in a music video featuring all of her family and the wedding guests. The look on her face was wonderful!

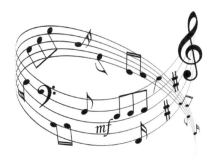

TV presenter

Moon River

My song is 'Moon River'. I think the original is by Andy Williams, but I love when Audrey Hepburn sings it in *Breakfast at Tiffany's*. I adore it, the song makes me cry and conveys so much emotion. I don't think there is another song so timeless and moving.

Screenwriter and film director

Brownsville Girl by Bob Dylan

There are so many songs that make me cry – I thought I'd pick a song that always makes me laugh.

There are a few of them – I always love that moment in 'Baker Street', where Gerry Rafferty sings – 'I can't say no – no, no, no, no, no, no, no.' He's lying – he can say 'no' – lots of times. But a song that is deliberately funny, and always makes me chuckle is 'Brownsville Girl' by Bob Dylan. Hard to imagine a life without Dylan – such a constant companion, in joy and sorrow. It's really long, Brownsville Girl – 11 minutes and God alone knows what it's about – but it contains these two wonderful lines – " The only thing we knew for sure about Henry Porter is that his name wasn't Henry Porter – and you know there was something about you baby I liked that was always too good for this world – just like you always said there was something about me you liked that I left in the French Quarter."

I never really feel like putting on a Dylan album – but when I do, I'm always happy.

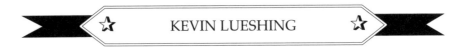

Professional boxer (former British welter weight champion and I.B.O welter weight world champion)

All I Do Is Think About You by Stevie Wonder

My special song is 'All I Do is Think About You' by Stevie Wonder as it reminds me of a lady who is so gorgeous.

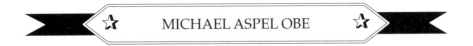

MICHAEL ASPEL OBE

TV presenter

The Way You Look Tonight by Fred Astaire

I would choose 'The Way You Look Tonight' sung by Fred Astaire, which always conjures up visions of my mother in a blue dress, about to go out for the evening. She didn't go out a lot, so it must have been a special occasion. Anyway, I love the song and have done since childhood.

Manager of Belfast Giants Ice Hockey Team

Galway Girl

I will always remember the first time I heard 'Galway Girl'. It was Christmas Eve in 2001 in a little bar in Belfast called Fibber Magee's. Being from Canada, we knew we couldn't fly home for Christmas, so what was expected to be a lonely Christmas ended up as one of my favourite Christmas memories. The song was such a hit with everyone in Fibber's that night that the band must have played it a dozen times, letting everyone and anyone from the crowd get up and sing it with them. To this day when I hear that song, which in Ireland is quite often, it reminds me of my first Christmas in Belfast, old men dancing while holding pints of Guinness on their heads, arm in arm with complete strangers not knowing the words, but belting out the chorus a dozen times.

WENDY HOLDEN

Novelist and journalist

Diamonds Are a Girl's Best Friend

'Diamonds Are A Girl's Best Friend' always conjures up for me driving along the Grande Corniche in the South of France with my husband. It was years ago and we only had a tape, but the witty lyrics and the general glamour of the song never fail to bring back the great fun we had, and continue to have in what is for us a very special place. The Riviera has become hugely over-visited and over-developed since we first started going a quarter century ago, but the beauty is still there if you know where to look. The other thing about this song is the sheer inventive dynamism and esprit of the words; so few songs are funny as this one is and it speaks of a more sophisticated era. I never got any diamonds though – we had no money then and even now I would hate to be bought them in case, as is likely, I lost them!

DJ and former professional rugby league player

Waiting for You by Dina Vass

The song that evokes the best memories for me is a song called, 'Waiting for You' by Dina Vass – Soul Avengers remix. It's the reason why I decided to learn to DJ as I just loved the effect that playing a particular song could have on a crowd of people, uniting their euphoria. Since retiring from professional sport DJing and music has become my number one passion. That song always brings back many happy memories of fun times on the island of Ibiza.

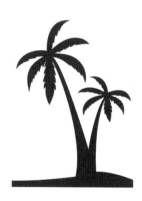

Playwright, screenwriter and author

On Sundays, Aunt Eveline comes over from Bradford and there are musical evenings at Gilpin Place. The children are warned to keep back as a shovelful of burning coals from the kitchen range is carried smoking through the house to light the fire in the sitting room, before we sit down to high tea in the kitchen. After tea, we all adjourn and, the sitting room still smelling of smoke, Aunt Eveline arranges herself at the piano stool and with my father on the violin (Now then, Walter, what shall we give them?) kicks off with a selection from 'Glamorous Night'. Then, having played themselves in, they accompany Uncle George, my father's brother, in some songs. Uncle George is a bricklayer and has a fine voice and a face as red as his bricks. He sings 'Bless this House' and 'Where'er You Walk', and sometimes Grandma has a little cry.

(Taken from 'Telling Tales' with kind permission from Alan Bennett.)

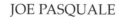

JOE PASQUALE

Comedian and TV star

Battle of Britain theme

One of my passions, if that is the right word, is flying. I have a Private Pilot's Licence and one of the reasons I wanted to fly was after seeing the film *The Battle of Britain* as a lad. I'd wished then that I could have been a fighter pilot. So every time I hear the theme tune to the film *The Battle of Britain*, it brings me back those days of wishful thinking as a boy.

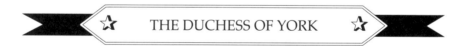

THE DUCHESS OF YORK

This Guy's in Love With You by Herb Alpert

'This Guy's in Love with You' by Herb Albert. This was her mother's favourite song and every time The Duchess hears it, she thinks of her.

Singer songwriter

Hey Ya by OutKast

I found this assignment quite hard as I remember so many evocative songs, lots of them sad, transporting me back to first crushes, relationships ending, even death. Then there are songs from the fashions and phases in my life like Disco and Northern Soul where I would obsess about a song and bust my moves. I was already perfecting and performing down the local club even before it had occurred to me to start singing. Music is a powerful backdrop to our lives. I have, however, decided to pick an upbeat, quite recent song – 'Hey Ya' by OutKast. My son Dylan was 13 months old in September 2003, 'Hey Ya' was riding high in the charts and on heavy rotation on the radio. Every time he heard it, he would stand on the dining room chair or grab anything to help him stand up, stick his bum out and bounce his nappy up and down vigorously shouting 'Ice Cold!'. It has become known as Dylan's nappy song. A born performer; watch out, the next generation is coming!

TV and weather presenter

State of Independence by Chrissie Hynde

The first time I heard 'State of Independence' was at a party back in the early eighties It was the Donna Summer version and the tune stayed in my head. I remember dancing that balmy midsummer night away, surrounded by friends and thinking that this inspiring song, played time and time again at the party, summed up just how happy I felt. Then, about ten years later, I heard the Chrissie Hynde version at the end of the film *Single White Female* and it blew my mind away. I watched the credits till the screen turned to black and vowed to move heaven and earth till I got a copy of the soundtrack of the film. It's from the first album by Moodswings. Moodfood is all very kick back and relax stuff, and on one of three tracks called Spiritual High, Chrissie Hynde from the Pretenders sings 'State of Independence', with Martin Luther King's speech 'I Have a Dream' overlapping the music at the end – a real uplifting, poignant and powerful touch. And to cap it all, when I got home the night I first met my soon to be husband at a Whitehall function, I switched on the radio, and my spine tingled ... there was Chrissie Hynde's beautiful voice singing:

"Love like a signal you call

Touching my body my soul"

Comedian, actor, musician

What Do You Wanna Make Those Eyes at Me For by Emile Ford and the Checkmates

When I was young and first started playing drums, one of my favourite songs I used to play along with on my drumkit was by Emile Ford called 'What do you wanna make those eyes at me for'. Happy memories.

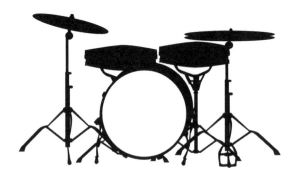

Actor

Oh Yes, I Remember it Well

The song that brings most memories is 'Oh Yes, I Remember it Well'. It was written by Alan J Lerner for the musical *Gigi* and recalls some of the best times of my professional life. While rehearsing for the first revival of *My Fair Lady* in London we were directed by Alan and he subsequently became a very dear friend. 'I Remember it Well' is a lovely funny duet with two aged lovers trying to remember their last evening together. He gets it all wrong (of course) and she gets it all right. I have performed it a couple of times, firstly with Liz Robertson, Alan Lerner's widow, at a charity evening, and again with June Whitfield, another old friend, at a musical gala.

Actress

When I'm Calling You by Nelson Eddy

When my brother Allistair and I were taken out in the car for family outings my father used to sing to us, and we would join in, singing lustily and allowing Daddy to have his solo moments. One of the songs I remember best was 'When I'm Calling You' we loved to warble the 'oooh-oooh-oooh' at the end of each line.

I sometimes hear it on the radio recorded by Nelson Eddy, and I'm filled with longing for my childhood and my beloved Mum and Dad.

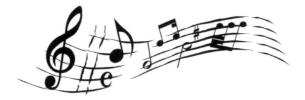

Novelist, musician

The utter impossibility of declaring a song your favourite, or an artist, or a composer, perhaps ranks with the similar utter impossibility of naming your favourite book or author. Art – of any form – is an aesthetic concept. It is a wavelength, it is an emotion, it is a feeling. We love books that others loathe. We are captivated by music that others fail to comprehend at all.

I was asked in a magazine interview a couple of weeks ago to list the first ten songs that appeared on my iPod if set to shuffle. What did I find? I found Shostakovich, followed by 'The Sir Douglas Quintet', followed by 'The Thirteenth Floor Elevators', 'The Cramps', 'The Gun Club, 'Suzanne Vega', 'Son House', 'Leadbelly', 'Simon and Garfunkel', 'Holst', and 'Little Feat'. A disparate and motley assortment of seemingly unrelated artistes.

But no. Perhaps not.

With me, the most important thing about any novel is the emotion it evokes. The reason for writing about the subjects I do is simply that such subjects give me the greatest opportunity to write about real people and how they deal with real situations. There is nothing in life more interesting than people, and one of the most interesting aspects of people is their ability to overcome difficulty and survive. I think I write 'human dramas', and in those dramas I feel I have sufficient canvas to paint the whole spectrum of human emotions, and this is what captures my attention. I once heard that non-fiction possesses, as its primary purpose, the conveying of information, whereas fiction possesses the primary purpose of evoking an emotion in the reader. I love writers that make me feel something – an emotion, whatever it might be – but I want to feel something as I read the book. There are millions of great books out there, all of them written very well, but they are mechanical in their plotting and style. Three weeks after reading them you might not recall anything about them. The books that really get me are the ones I remember months later. I might not recall the names of the characters or the intricacies of the plot, but I remember how it made me feel. For me, that's all important. The emotional connection.

And so it is with music.

I am a writer, first and foremost. But I am also a musician. I have always played a musical instrument. As a child it was the trumpet – everything from strident Souza Marches to Scott Joplin to Haydn Concertos. And now? Now I play guitar, even have a band, and I play rhythm 'n' blues, jazz, rock 'n' roll. But still – for me – it is all about the emotional connection.

I can cry because of a piece of music. A piece of music can make me serious, pensive, joyful, enthusiastic. I listen to music everywhere I go. I carry my iPod, loaded up with the better part of four thousand songs and compositions, and my life has a soundtrack. At home I cook for the family in a large kitchen, and the stereo is there in the kitchen, and there are six or seven hundreds CDs to choose from, and sometimes I want to listen to five or six or ten at once. But no matter the circumstances, there is always music. Always has been.

Just as books can create and end friendships, so can music. So much the case in social networks these days, people connect because of similar tastes in music. What are they saying? There's a damned good possibility we will get along because we can relate to the same music, the same emotions, the same gut responses. I believe that music is not only the food of love, but the food of life.

And I have found so many authors are themselves musicians, and I wonder if there is a rhythm in music than can also be found in words. I certainly believe so. Paragraphs are like passages, words like notes, and often I will read something back after I've written it and feel that there is one too many syllables. I change a word, I remove that extra beat, and the rhythm feels right. That's just the way I am, the way I work, and though that may be strange it is nevertheless what I feel.

And so it is – when asked to name a favourite song, a favourite composer, a favourite band – it is not possible to give an answer. There is no favourite, and what may be special today is overtaken by something more special tomorrow.

Gustav Mahler said, 'If a composer could say what he had to say in words he would not bother trying to say it in music'. There are many ills in life – of the spirit, the mind, the body, the heart. All of them had found their remedy somewhere in music, if only for the listener to feel that there is some other human being who has experienced what they themselves have experienced.

As John Logan so famously said, 'Music is the medicine of the mind'

And so it is. I have no favourite. I have no song or psalm or concerto or symphony that stands above other by head or shoulders.

I just have my love of music, and that is enough for me.